Medi
Pocke
Refer   W9-CIJ-289

DRUGS
2005

Medical
Pocket
Reference

DRUGS
2005

LIPPINCOTT WILLIAMS & WILKINS
A **Wolters Kluwer** Company

Philadelphia • Baltimore • New York • London
Buenos Aires • Hong Kong • Sydney • Tokyo

Staff

Publisher
Judith A. Schilling McCann, RN, MSN

Editorial Director
William J. Kelly

Clinical Director
Joan M. Robinson, RN, MSN

Senior Art Director
Arlene Putterman

Art Director
Elaine Kasmer

Clinical Manager
Eileen Cassin Gallen, RN, BSN

Drug Information Editor
Melissa M. Devlin, PharmD

Editorial Project Manager
Christiane L. Brownell

Clinical Project Manager
Minh N. Luu, RN, BSN, JD

Editor
Lynne Christensen

Clinical Editor
Lisa M. Bonsall, RN, MSN, CRNP

Copy Editor
Jenifer F. Walker

Digital Composition Services
Diane Paluba (manager),
Joyce Rossi Biletz, Donald G. Knauss

Manufacturing
Patricia K. Dorshaw (director),
Beth J. Welsh

Editorial Assistants
Carol A. Caputo, Tara L. Carter-Bell

Indexer
Dianne Prewitt

Visit our Web site at eDrugInfo.com

ISBN 1-58255-345-9
ISSN 1531-4308
MPRD05—D N O S A J J M A M F J
06 05 10 9 8 7 6 5 4 3 2

Contents

How to use this book

Medical Pocket Reference: Drugs 2005 is designed to help you find essential drug information quickly. A list of all the abbreviations used in the drug entries appears first. The entries are organized alphabetically by generic name. Under each generic name, you'll find common brand names. Canadian brand names are followed by an asterisk (*).

Each drug entry then shows the drug's pharmacologic class and (after the semicolon) the therapeutic class. Next is the pregnancy risk category and, where applicable, controlled substance schedule.

Next is information about the drug's available forms—the drug's preparations and dosage strengths.

The last section of the drug entries covers major indications and the most common dosages ordered. In this section, the multiplication symbol ($\times$) is used for the word *for* to save space. The following symbols indicate when dosage adjustments are needed for renally impaired (†), hepatically impaired (‡), immunocompromised (§), and debilitated patients (¶).

One new appendix describes the meaning of Pregnancy Risk Categories, and another explains the Controlled Substance Schedule. Other appendices list drugs whose levels are reduced by dialysis, drugs that prolong the QTc interval, rates of infusion for common drugs, and dangerous laboratory test values and their possible causes.

The index covers trade names and indications.

Guide to abbreviations

ABG	arterial blood gas	COPD	chronic obstructive pulmonary disease
ac	before meals	CrCl	creatinine clearance
ACE	angiotensin-converting enzyme	CSF	cerebrospinal fluid
ADHD	attention-deficit hyperactivity disorder	CSS	Controlled Substance Schedule
AIDS	acquired immunodeficiency syndrome	CV	cardiovascular
		CVA	cerebrovascular accident
ALL	acute lymphocytic leukemia	CYP	cytochrome P450
ALT	alanine aminotransferase	d	day
am	before noon	dl	deciliter
APTT	activated partial thromboplastin time	DM	diabetes mellitus
		DVT	deep vein thrombosis
ASAP	as soon as possible	D_5W	dextrose 5% in water
AST	aspartate aminotransferase	ET	endotracheal
bid	twice a day	exam	examination
BM	bowel movement	g	gram
BP	blood pressure	GERD	gastroesophageal reflux disease
BPH	benign prostatic hyperplasia		
		GGT	gamma-glutamyl transpeptidase
BUN	blood urea nitrogen		
CA	cancer	GI	gastrointestinal
CAD	coronary artery disease	gram-neg	gram-negative
CBC	complete blood count	gram-pos	gram-positive
cGMP	cyclic guanosine monophosphate	GU	genitourinary
		GYN	gynecologic
chemo	chemotherapy	H	histamine
cm	centimeter	HbA_{1c}	glycosylated hemoglobin
CMV	cytomegalovirus		

HBV	hepatitis B virus	MAC	*Mycobacterium avium* complex
Hct	hematocrit		
HDL	high-density lipoprotein	MAO	monoamine oxidase
HF	heart failure	max	maximum
Hgb	hemoglobin	mcg	microgram
HIV	human immunodeficiency virus	mEq	milliequivalent
		mg	milligram
HMG-CoA	3-hydroxy-3-methylglutaryl coenzyme A	MI	myocardial infarction
		min	minute
H_2O	water	ml	milliliter
hr	hour	mo	month
hs	at bedtime	MS	multiple sclerosis
HSV	herpes simplex virus	NaCl	sodium chloride
HTN	hypertension	ng	nanogram
IBS	irritable bowel syndrome	NG	nasogastric
IM	intramuscular	NSAID	nonsteroidal anti-inflammatory drug
INR	international normalized ratio		
		NSS	normal saline solution
intraop	intraoperative	OA	osteoarthritis
IOP	intraocular pressure	OCD	obsessive-compulsive disorder
IPPB	intermittent positive-pressure breathing		
		OM	otitis media
IU	international unit	oz	ounce
IV	intravenous	PAC	premature atrial contraction
kg	kilogram	PAT	paroxysmal atrial tachycardia
L	liter		
LDH	lactate dehydrogenase	pc	after meals
LDL	low-density lipoprotein	PCN	penicillin
liq	liquid	PDE5	phosphodiesterase type 5
m^2	square meter	PE	pulmonary embolism
		periop	perioperative

PID	pelvic inflammatory disease	ST	sinus tachycardia
pm	after noon	staph	staphylococci
PMDD	premenstrual dysphoric disorder	strep	streptococci
PO	by mouth	SVT	supraventricular tachycardia
postop	postoperative	TB	tuberculosis
PR	by rectum	tbs	tablespoon
PRC	pregnancy risk category	TCA	tricyclic antidepressant
preop	preoperative	temp	temperature
prn	as needed	tid	three times a day
PSVT	paroxysmal supraventricular tachycardia	TSH	thyroid-stimulating hormone
PT	prothrombin time	tsp	teaspoon
PTT	partial thromboplastin time	UTI	urinary tract infection
PVC	premature ventricular contraction	VF	ventricular fibrillation
PVT	paroxysmal ventricular tachycardia	VT	ventricular tachycardia
		WBC	white blood cell
q	every	WHO	World Health Organization
qid	four times a day	wk	week
RA	rheumatoid arthritis	wkly	weekly
RBC	red blood cell	wt	weight
RDA	recommended dietary allowance	yr	year
RF	renal failure		
RNA	ribonucleic acid		
SC	subcutaneous		
sec	second		
SL	sublingual		
SSRI	selective serotonin reuptake inhibitor		

abacavir sulfate
Ziagen

Nucleoside analogue reverse transcriptase inhibitor; antiretroviral
PRC: C

Available forms
Oral solution: 20 mg/ml; *Tablets:* 300 mg

Indications & dosages
➤ *HIV-1 infection*—**Adult:** 300 mg PO bid with other antiretrovirals. **Child 3 mo-16 yr:** 8 mg/kg PO bid; max, 300 mg with other antiretrovirals.

acarbose
Precose

Alpha-glucosidase inhibitor; antidiabetic
PRC: B

Available forms
Tablets: 50, 100 mg

Indications & dosages
➤ *Type 2 DM, adjunct to insulin or metformin in type 2 DM*—**Adult:** 25 mg PO tid with main meal; adjust q 4-8 wk. Maintenance, 50-100 mg PO tid. Max, 50 mg tid for patients ≤ 60 kg and 100 mg tid for patients > 60 kg.

acetaminophen (APAP, paracetamol)
Acephen, Aceta, Anacin (aspirin free), Apacet, Feverall, Genapap Children's, Neopap, Panadol, Tempra, Tylenol

Para-aminophenol derivative; nonopioid analgesic, antipyretic
PRC: B

Available forms
Caplets: 160, 500 mg; *Caplets (extended-release):* 650 mg; *Capsules:* 325, 500 mg; *Elixir:* 80 mg/2.5 ml, 80 mg/5 ml, 120 mg/5 ml, 160 mg/5 ml; *Gelcaps:* 500 mg; *Liq:* 160 mg/5 ml, 500 mg/5 ml; *Oral liq:* 160 mg/5 ml, 500 mg/15 ml; *Oral solution:* 48, 100 mg/ml; *Sprinkle:* 80, 160 mg/capsule; *Suppository:* 80, 120, 125, 300, 325, 650 mg; *Tablets:* 160, 325, 500, 650 mg; *Tablets (chewable):* 80 mg

Indications & dosages
➤ *Pain, fever*—**Adult, child > 11 yr:** 325-650 mg PO q 4-6 hr prn; or 1 g PO tid or qid prn. Or, 2 extended-release capsules PO q 8 hr. Max, 4 g daily. For long-term, max 2.6 g daily. **Child 11 yr:** 480 mg PO q 4-6 hr prn. **Child 9-10 yr:** 400 mg PO q 4-6 hr prn. **Child 6-8 yr:** 320 mg PO q 4-6 hr prn. **Child 4-5 yr:** 240 mg PO q 4-6 hr prn. **Child 2-3 yr:** 160 mg PO q 4-6 hr prn. **Child 12-23 mo:** 120 mg PO q 4-6 hr prn. **Child 4-11 mo:** 80 mg PO q 4-6 hr prn. **Child ≤ 3 mo:** 40 mg PO q 4-6 hr prn.
PR dosing. **Child 6-12 yr:** 325 mg PR q 4-6 hr prn. Max, 2.6 g in 14 hr. **Child 3-6 yr:** 120-125 mg PR q 4-6 hr prn. Max, 720 mg in 24 hr. **Child 1-3 yr:** 80 mg PR

---

§ Adjust in immunocompromised patients　　　¶ Adjust in debilitated patients

q 4 hr prn. **Child 3-11 mo:** 80 mg PR q 6 hr prn.

acetylcysteine
Acetadote, Mucomyst, Mucosil-10, Mucosil-20

Amino acid (L-cysteine) derivative; mucolytic, antidote for acetaminophen overdose
PRC: B

Available forms
Injection: 20% solution in 30-ml single-dose vials; *Solution:* 10%, 20%

Indications & dosages
➤ *Thick mucous secretions*—**Adult, child:** 1-2 ml of 10% or 20% solution by direct instillation into trachea q 1 hr prn; or 1-10 ml of 20% solution or 2-20 ml of 10% solution by nebulizer q 2-6 hr prn.
➤ *Acetaminophen toxicity*—**Adult, child:** 140 mg/kg PO; then 70 mg/kg PO q 4 hr × 17 doses. Or, 150 mg/kg IV in 200 ml D₅W over 15 min as loading dose, then maintenance of 50 mg/kg IV in 500 ml D₅W over 4 hr followed by 100 mg/kg IV in 1L of D₅W over 16 hr.

activated charcoal
Actidose, Actidose-Aqua, CharcoAid, CharcoAid 2000, CharcoCaps, Liqui-Char

Adsorbent; antidote, antidiarrheal, antiflatulent
PRC: C

Available forms
Capsules: 260 mg; *Oral suspension:* 12.5, 15, 25, 30, 50 g; *Powder:* 15, 30, 40, 120, 240 g; *Tablets:* 250 mg

Indications & dosages
➤ *Flatulence, dyspepsia*—**Adult:** 600 mg-5 g PO in 1 dose or 0.975-3.9 g PO tid pc.
➤ *Poisoning*—**Adult, child:** 1-2 g/kg (30-100 g) PO or 10 times the amount of poison ingested; give as suspension in 120-240 ml H₂O. Give within 30 min of ingestion of poison.

acyclovir sodium
Avirax*, Zovirax

Synthetic purine nucleoside; antiviral
PRC: C

Available forms
Capsules: 200 mg; *Injection:* 500 mg, 1-g/vial; *Suspension:* 200 mg/5 ml; *Tablets:* 400, 800 mg

Indications & dosages
➤ *Mucocutaneous HSV infection in immunocompromised patients; genital herpes in immunocompetent patients*—**Adult, child ≥ 12 yr:** 5 mg/kg IV q 8 hr × 7 d. **Child < 12 yr:** 250 mg/m² IV q 8 hr × 7 d.†
➤ *Initial genital herpes*—**Adult:** 200 mg PO q 4 hr while awake (total 5 capsules daily); or 400 mg PO q 8 hr. Continue 7-10 d.†
➤ *Recurrent genital herpes*—**Adult:** 400 mg PO bid ≤ 12 mo.†
➤ *Varicella infection in immunocompromised patients*—**Adult, child ≥ 12 yr:**

10 mg/kg IV q 8 hr × 7 d. **Child < 12 yr:**
20 mg/kg IV q 8 hr × 7 d.†

adalimumab
Humira

Monoclonal antibody; antiarthritic
PRC: B

Available forms
Injection: 40-mg/ml vial; *Prefilled syringe:*
40 mg/ml

Indications & dosages
➤ *To reduce signs and symptoms and inhibit progression of structural damage in
patients with moderate to severe RA who
haven't responded to disease-modifying
antirheumatics or methotrexate—***Adult:**
40 mg SC q other wk. Patients not taking
methotrexate may benefit with 40 mg
q wk.

adefovir dipivoxil
Hepsera

Acyclic nucleotide analogue; antiviral
PRC: C

Available forms
Tablets: 10 mg

Indications & dosages
➤ *Chronic hepatitis B—***Adult:** 10 mg PO
daily.†

adenosine
Adenocard

Nucleoside; antiarrhythmic
PRC: C

Available forms
Injection: 3 mg/ml in 2-ml vials, 2-ml
syringes, 5-ml syringes

Indications & dosages
➤ *PSVT—***Adult:** 6 mg rapid IV push
over 1-2 sec. If PSVT persists after 1-
2 min, 12 mg by rapid IV push; repeat
12-mg dose once prn.

albuterol (salbutamol)
Proventil, Ventolin

albuterol sulfate
(salbutamol sulfate)
AccuNeb, Proventil, Proventil HFA,
Proventil Repetabs, Ventolin, Ventolin
HFA, Volmax

Adrenergic; bronchodilator
PRC: C

Available forms
albuterol *Aerosol inhalation:* 90 mcg/
metered spray; **albuterol sulfate** *Solution
(for inhalation):* 0.083%, 0.5%, 0.63 mg/
3 ml, 1.25 mg/3 ml; *Syrup:* 2 mg/5 ml;
Tablets: 2, 4 mg; *Tablets (extended-
release):* 4, 8 mg

Indications & dosages
➤ *Bronchospasm—***Adult, child ≥ 12 yr:**
1 or 2 inhalations aerosol inhalant q 4-
6 hr. Or, 2.5 mg solution for inhalation tid

---

or qid by nebulizer. Or, 2-4 mg tablets PO tid or qid; max, 8 mg qid. Or, 4-8 mg extended-release PO q 12 hr; max, 16 mg bid. **Child 6-12 yr:** 2 mg (1 tsp) PO tid or qid. **Child 2-6 yr:** 0.1 mg/kg PO tid up to 0.2 mg/kg tid; max, 4 mg tid. **Adult > 65 yr:** 2 mg PO tid or qid.
➤ *Prevention of exercise-induced bronchospasm*—**Adult, child ≥ 4 yr:** 2 inhalations 15 min before exercise.

alefacept
Amevive

Immunosuppressant; antipsoriatic
PRC: B

Available forms
I.M. injection: 15-mg single-dose vial

Indications & dosages
➤ *Moderate to severe chronic plaque psoriasis in candidates for systemic therapy or phototherapy*—
Adult: 15 mg IM q wk × 12 wk. If CD4+ T lymphocyte count is normal and ≥ 12 wk since the previous treatment, may give another 12-wk course.§

alendronate sodium
Fosamax

Osteoclast-mediated bone resorption inhibitor; antiosteoporotic
PRC: C

Available forms
Tablets: 5, 10, 35, 40, 70 mg

Indications & dosages
➤ *Osteoporosis in postmenopausal women; to increase bone mass in men with osteoporosis*—**Adult:** 10 mg PO daily or 70-mg tablet PO q wk with full glass of H_2O only, ≥ 30 min before 1st food, liq, or drug of day.
➤ *Prevention of osteoporosis in postmenopausal women*—**Woman:** 5 mg PO daily or 35-mg tablet PO q wk with full glass of H_2O only, ≥ 30 min before 1st food, liq, or drug of day.
➤ *Corticosteroid-induced osteoporosis*—**Adult:** 5 mg PO daily with full glass of H_2O only, ≥ 30 min before 1st food, liq, or drug of day. In postmenopausal women not receiving estrogen replacement therapy, 10 mg PO daily.
➤ *Paget's disease of bone*—**Adult:** 40 mg PO daily × 6 mo with full glass of H_2O only, ≥ 30 min before 1st food, liq, or drug of day.

alfuzosin hydrochloride
Uroxatral

Selective alpha$_1$-adrenoreceptor antagonist; BPH drug
PRC: B

Available forms
Tablets (extended-release): 10 mg

Indications & dosages
➤ *BPH*—**Man:** 10 mg PO right after the same meal q d.

---

allopurinol
Apo-Allopurinol*, Zyloprim

allopurinol sodium
Aloprim

Xanthine oxidase inhibitor; antigout drug
PRC: C

Available forms
Powder for injection: 500 mg/3 ml;
Tablets (scored): 100, 300 mg

Indications & dosages
➤ *Gout or hyperuricemia*—May be given as single dose or divided, but divide doses > 300 mg. **Adult:** Mild gout, 200-300 mg PO daily; severe gout with large tophi, 400-600 mg PO daily. Max, 800 mg/d.†
➤ *Hyperuricemia caused by malignancies*—**Adult, child > 10 yr:** 200-400 mg/m^2/d IV as a single infusion or equally divided dose q 6, 8, or 12 hr. Max, 600 mg/d.† **Child ≤ 10 yr:** Initially, 200 mg/m^2/d IV as single infusion or equally divided dose q 6, 8, or 12 hr. Titrate according to uric acid level. Or, for child 6-10 yr, 300 mg PO daily or divide tid; for child < 6 yr, 150 mg PO daily.†
➤ *To prevent acute gout attacks*—**Adult:** 100 mg PO daily; increase at wkly intervals by 100 mg to max 800 mg/d until uric acid level falls to ≤ 6 mg/dl.†
➤ *To prevent uric acid nephropathy during CA chemo*—**Adult:** 600-800 mg PO daily for 2 or 3 d, with high fluid intake.†
➤ *Recurrent calcium oxalate calculi*—**Adult:** 200-300 mg PO daily as a single dose or in divided doses.†

almotriptan
Axert

Serotonin-1 receptor agonist; anti-migraine drug
PRC: C

Available forms
Tablets: 6.25, 12.5 mg

Indications & dosages
➤ *Acute migraine with or without aura*—**Adult:** 6.25- or 12.5-mg tablet PO, with 1 additional dose after 2 hr if headache is unresolved or recurs. Max, 2 doses/24 hr.‡

alosetron hydrochloride
Lotronex

Selective 5-HT$_3$ receptor antagonist; anti-IBS drug
PRC: B

Available forms
Tablets: 1 mg

Indications & dosages
➤ *IBS in women who have had chronic symptoms for ≥ 6 mo, who have no GI tract abnormalities, and who don't respond to conventional therapy*—**Woman:** 1 mg PO daily. Increase dose to 1 mg bid, prn, after 4 wk. If adequate control isn't reached after 4 wk on bid therapy, stop drug.

---

§ Adjust in immunocompromised patients

¶ Adjust in debilitated patients

alprazolam
Apo-Alpraz*, Novo-Alprazol*,
Nu-Alpraz*, Xanax, Xanax XR

Benzodiazepine; anxiolytic
PRC: D; CSS: IV

Available forms
Oral solution: 0.5 mg/5 ml, 1 mg/ml (concentrate); *Tablets:* 0.25, 0.5, 1, 2 mg; *Tablets (extended-release):* 0.5, 1, 2, 3 mg

Indications & dosages
➤ *Anxiety*—**Adult:** 0.25-0.5 mg PO tid. Max, 4 mg daily in divided doses. **Elderly or debilitated patient, patient with advanced liver disease:** Initially, 0.25 mg PO bid or tid. Max, 4 mg daily in divided doses.
➤ *Panic disorders*—**Adult:** 0.5 mg PO tid; increase q 3 or 4 d in increments of 1 mg/d. Max, 10 mg daily in divided doses. Or, initially 0.5-1 mg extended-release PO daily; increase q 3 or 4 d in increments of 1 mg/d. Max, 10 mg/d.

alteplase (tissue plasminogen activator, recombinant; t-PA)
Activase, Cathflo Activase

Enzyme; thrombolytic enzyme
PRC: C

Available forms
Injection: 50-, 100-mg vials; 2-ml vials for intracatheter instillation

Indications & dosages
➤ *Lysis of thrombi in acute MI*—**Adult ≥ 65 kg:** 60 mg IV in 1st hr (6-10 mg as bolus over 1st 1-2 min). Then 20 mg/hr × 2 hr. **Adult < 65 kg:** 0.75 mg/kg IV in 1st hr (0.045-0.075 mg/kg as bolus over 1st 1-2 min). Then, 0.25 mg/kg/hr × 2 hr.
➤ *PE*—**Adult:** 100 mg IV over 2 hr. Begin heparin at end of infusion when PTT or thrombin time returns to ≤ 2 times normal.
➤ *Acute ischemic stroke*—**Adult:** 0.9 mg/kg IV over 1 hr with 10% of total dose given as initial IV bolus over 1st min. Give within 3 hr of start of symptoms and after intracranial bleeding is ruled out. Max, 90 mg.
➤ *Restoration of function to central venous access device*—**Adult, child > 2 yr:** For patients > 30 kg, instill 2 mg in 2 ml sterile H_2O into catheter. For patients 10-30 kg, instill 110% of the catheter's internal lumen volume. Max, 2 mg. After 30 min of dwell time, assess catheter function by aspirating blood. If function is restored, aspirate and discard 4-5 ml of blood, then gently flush catheter with NSS. If function isn't restored after 2 hr, repeat dose.

amantadine hydrochloride
Symadine, Symmetrel

Synthetic cyclic primary amine; antiviral, antiparkinsonian
PRC: C

Available forms
Capsules: 100 mg; *Syrup:* 50 mg/5 ml; *Tablets:* 100 mg

Indications & dosages

➤ *Influenza type A virus*—Start ASAP after exposure, preferably 24-48 hr after symptoms appear. Continue × 24-48 hr after they disappear. **Adult ≤ 65 yr, child ≥ 13 yr:** 200 mg PO daily in 1 dose or divided bid.† **Child 9-12 yr:** 100 mg PO bid.†
Child 1-8 yr: 4.4-8.8 mg/kg PO daily in 1 dose or divided bid, to 150 mg daily.†
Adult > 65 yr: 100 mg PO daily.†
➤ *Parkinson's disease*—**Adult:** 100 mg PO bid. For patients on other antiparkinsonians or seriously ill patients, 100 mg PO daily × 1-2 wk; then 100 mg PO bid. Max, 400 mg/d.†

amifostine
Ethyol

Organic thiophosphate; cytoprotective drug
PRC: C

Available forms
Injection: 500 mg anhydrous base

Indications & dosages

➤ *Reduction of renal toxicity with repeated cisplatin administration in patients with advanced ovarian or non–small-cell lung CA*—**Adult:** 910 mg/m² daily as 15 min IV infusion, starting 30 min before chemo. If hypotension occurs and BP is abnormal ≤ 5 min after treatment stops, use 740 mg/m² for subsequent cycles.
➤ *Xerostomia in patients having postop radiation for head or neck CA*—**Adult:** 200 mg/m² daily as 3-min IV infusion, starting 15-30 min before radiation.

amikacin sulfate
Amikin

Aminoglycoside; antibiotic
PRC: D

Available forms
Injection: 50, 250 mg/ml

Indications & dosages

➤ *Serious infection*—**Adult, child:** 15 mg/kg/d divided q 8-12 hr by IM or IV infusion.† **Neonate:** Loading dose, 10 mg/kg IV; then, 7.5 mg/kg q 12 hr.†
➤ *Uncomplicated UTI*—**Adult:** 250 mg IM or IV bid.†

aminophylline (theophylline ethylenediamine)
Phyllocontin, Truphylline

Xanthine derivative; bronchodilator
PRC: C

Available forms
Injection: 250 mg/10 ml; 500 mg/20 ml; *Oral liq:* 105 mg/ml; *Rectal suppository:* 250, 500 mg; *Tablets:* 100, 200 mg; *Tablets (controlled-release):* 225 mg; *Tablets (extended-release):* 350 mg*

Indications & dosages

➤ *Bronchospasm*—**Patient not taking theophylline:** Loading dose, 6 mg/kg IV; then maintenance infusion. **Adult (nonsmoker) not taking theophylline:** 0.7 mg/

---

§ Adjust in immunocompromised patients   ¶ Adjust in debilitated patients

kg/hr IV × 12 hr; then 0.5 mg/kg/hr. **Otherwise healthy adult smoker not taking theophylline:** 1 mg/kg/hr IV × 12 hr; then 0.8 mg/kg/hr. **Child 9-16 yr not taking theophylline:** 1 mg/kg/hr IV × 12 hr; then 0.8 mg/kg/hr. **Child 6 mo-9 yr not taking theophylline:** 1.2 mg/kg/hr × 12 hr; then 1 mg/kg/hr. **Patient taking theophylline:** Infuse 0.63 mg/kg to increase drug level by 1 mcg/ml. If no sign of toxicity, 3.1 mg/kg.

➤ *Chronic bronchial asthma*—**Adult, child:** 16 mg/kg or 400 mg (whichever is less) PO daily in divided doses q 6-8 hr (for rapidly absorbed forms). May increase by 25% q 2-3 d. Or, 12 mg/kg or 400 mg (whichever is less) PO daily in divided doses q 8-12 hr (extended-release). May increase by 2-3 mg/kg/d q 3 d.

amiodarone hydrochloride
Cordarone, Pacerone

Benzofuran derivative; antiarrhythmic
PRC: D

Available forms
Injection: 50 mg/ml; *Tablets:* 200, 400 mg

Indications & dosages
➤ *Recurrent VF, unstable VT*—**Adult:** Loading dose, 800-1,600 mg PO daily × 1-3 wk until initial response; then 600-800 mg/d PO × 1 mo; maintenance, 200-600 mg PO daily. Or, loading, 150 mg IV over 10 min (15 mg/min); then 360 mg IV over next 6 hr (1 mg/min); then 540 mg IV over next 18 hr (0.5 mg/min). After 1st 24 hr, continue maintenance infusion of 720 mg/24 hr (0.5 mg/min).

amitriptyline hydrochloride
Apo-Amitriptyline*

TCA; antidepressant
PRC: D

Available forms
Injection: 10 mg/ml; *Tablets:* 10, 25, 50, 75, 100, 150 mg

Indications & dosages
➤ *Depression*—**Adult:** 50-100 mg PO hs; increase to 150 mg daily. Max, 300 mg daily prn. Maintenance, 50-100 mg/d PO or 20-30 mg IM qid. **Elderly, adolescent:** 10 mg PO tid plus 20 mg hs daily.

amlodipine besylate
Norvasc

Dihydropyridine calcium channel blocker; antianginal, antihypertensive
PRC: C

Available forms
Tablets: 2.5, 5, 10 mg

Indications & dosages
➤ *Angina*—**Adult:** 5-10 mg PO daily.
➤ *HTN*—**Adult:** Initially 2.5-5 mg PO daily. **Elderly:** 2.5 mg PO daily. For small or frail patients, patients using other antihypertensives, or those with hepatic insufficiency, start with 2.5 mg daily. Max, 10 mg/d. Adjust over 7-14 d. **Child ≥ 6 yr:** 2.5-5 mg PO daily.

amoxicillin and clavulanate potassium
Augmentin, Augmentin ES-600, Augmentin XR, Clavulin*

Aminopenicillin, beta-lactamase inhibitor; antibiotic
PRC: B

Available forms
Oral suspension: 125, 200, 250, 400, 600 mg amoxicillin trihydrate and 31.25, 28.5, 62.5, 57, 42.9 mg clavulanic acid, respectively, per 5 ml (after reconstitution); *Tablets (chewable):* 125, 200, 250, 400 mg amoxicillin trihydrate and 31.25, 28.5, 62.5, 57 mg clavulanic acid, respectively; *Tablets (extended-release):* 1,000 mg amoxicillin trihydrate/62.5 mg clavulanic acid; *Tablets (film-coated):* 250, 500, 875 mg amoxicillin trihydrate and 125, 125, 125 mg clavulanic acid, respectively

Indications & dosages
➤ *UTI; lower respiratory infection, OM, sinusitis, skin and skin-structure infection, from gram-pos and gram-neg organisms*—**Adult, child ≥ 40 kg:** 250-500 mg PO q 8 hr. **Child < 40 kg:** 20-40 mg/kg PO daily in divided doses q 8 hr.
➤ *Acute OM with antibiotic exposure ≤ 3 mo, in child ≤ 2 yr or in daycare*—**Child 3 mo-12 yr:** 90 mg/kg/d Augmentin ES-600 PO q 12 hr × 10 d.
➤ *Community-acquired pneumonia or acute bacterial sinusitis from confirmed or suspected beta-lactamase producing pathogens or Streptococcus pneumoniae with reduced susceptibility to penicillin*—

Adult, child ≥ 16 yr: 2,000 mg/125 mg (two extended-release tablets) q 12 hr × 7-10 d for pneumonia or 10 d for sinusitis.

amoxicillin trihydrate
Amoxil, Apo-Amoxi*, DisperMox, Novamoxin*, Nu-Amoxi*, Trimox

Aminopenicillin; antibiotic
PRC: B

Available forms
Capsules: 250, 500 mg; *Pediatric drops:* 50 mg/ml (after reconstitution); *Suspension:* 125 mg/5 ml, 200 mg/5 ml, 250 mg/5 ml, 400 mg/5 ml; *Tablets (chewable):* 200, 400 mg; *Tablets (film-coated):* 500, 875 mg; *Tablets (for oral suspension):* 200 mg, 400 mg

Indications & dosages
➤ *Mild to moderate infections of the ear, nose, or throat, skin and skin structure, GU tract*—**Adult:** 500 mg PO q 12 hr or 250 mg PO q 8 hr.† **Child > 3 mo:** 25 mg/kg/d in divided doses q 12 hr or 20 mg/kg/d in divided doses q 8 hr. **Neonates and infants ≤ 12 wk:** up to 30 mg/kg/d divided q 12 hr.
➤ *Severe infections of the ear, nose, or throat, skin and skin structure, GU tract; lower respiratory tract infection*—**Adult:** 875 mg PO q 12 hr or 500 mg PO q 8 hr.† **Child > 3 mo:** 45 mg/kg/d in divided doses q 12 hr or 40 mg/kg/d in divided doses q 8 hr. **Neonates and infants ≤ 12 wk:** Up to 30 mg/kg/d divided q 12 hr.
➤ *Uncomplicated gonorrhea*—**Adult:** 3 g PO.† **Prepubertal child ≥ 2 yr:** 50 mg/kg

§ Adjust in immunocompromised patients   ¶ Adjust in debilitated patients

amoxicillin combined with 25 mg/kg probenecid as a single dose.
➤ *Endocarditis prophylaxis for dental procedures*—**Adult:** 2 g PO in 1 dose 1 hr before procedure.† **Child > 2 yr:** 50 mg/kg PO in 1 dose 1 hr before procedure.
➤ *Chlamydia during pregnancy*—**Woman:** 500 mg/kg/d PO tid × 7-10 d.†

amphotericin B
Amphocin, Amphotericin B for Injection, Fungizone Intravenous

Polyene macrolide; antifungal
PRC: B

Available forms
Injection: 50-mg lyophilized cake

Indications & dosages
➤ *Fungal infection, meningitis*—**Adult:** Test dose of 1 mg in 20 ml D_5W infusion IV over 20-30 min. If tolerated, 0.25-0.3 mg/kg/d IV (0.1 mg/ml) over 2-6 hr. Increase gradually to max 1 mg/kg daily or 1.5 mg/kg q other d. If stopped for ≥ 1 wk, resume drug with initial dose and increase gradually.

amphotericin B cholesteryl sulfate complex
Amphotec

Polyene macrolide; antifungal
PRC: B

Available forms
Injection: 50 mg/20 ml, 100 mg/50 ml

Indications & dosages
➤ *Invasive aspergillosis in patient who doesn't respond to amphotericin B deoxycholate*—**Adult, child:** 3-4 mg/kg/d IV at 1 mg/kg/hr. Give test dose before starting treatment; infuse small amount (10 ml final preparation with 1.6-8.3 mg drug) over 15-30 min and monitor × next 30 min.

amphotericin B lipid complex
Abelcet

Polyene antibiotic; antifungal
PRC: B

Available forms
Suspension (for injection): 100 mg/20-ml vial

Indications & dosages
➤ *Invasive fungal infection in patient refractory to or intolerant of conventional amphotericin B therapy*—**Adult, child:** 5 mg/kg daily IV at 2.5 mg/kg/hr.

amphotericin B liposomal
AmBisome

Polyene antibiotic; antifungal
PRC: B

Available forms
Injection: 50-mg vial

Indications & dosages
➤ *Fungal infection in febrile, neutropenic patient*—**Adult, child:** 3 mg/kg IV infusion daily.

➤ *Systemic fungal infection in patient refractory to or intolerant of conventional amphotericin B treatment*—**Adult, child:** 3-5 mg/kg IV infusion daily.

➤ *Visceral leishmaniasis in immunocompetent patient*—**Adult, child:** 3 mg/kg IV infusion daily on d 1-5, 14, and 21. May repeat prn.

➤ *Visceral leishmaniasis in immunocompromised patient*—**Adult, child:** 4 mg/kg IV infusion daily on d 1-5, 10, 17, 24, 31, and 38.

➤ *Cryptococcal meningitis in HIV patient*—**Adult, child:** 6 mg/kg/d IV infusion over 2 hr. Infusion time may be reduced to 1 hr or increased prn.

---

ampicillin
Apo-Ampi*, Novo-Ampicillin*, Penbritin*

ampicillin sodium
Ampicin*, Penbritin*

ampicillin trihydrate
Principen

Aminopenicillin; antibiotic
PRC: B

Available forms
Capsules: 250, 500 mg; *Infusion:* 1, 2 g; *Injection:* 125, 250, 500 mg; 1, 2 g; *Suspension:* 125, 250 mg/5 ml (after reconstitution)

Indications & dosages
➤ *Systemic infection, UTI*—**Adult:** 250-500 mg PO q 6 hr.† **Child:** 50-100 mg/kg PO daily, in divided doses q 6 hr; or 100-200 mg/kg IM or IV daily, in divided doses q 6-8 hr.†

➤ *Bacterial meningitis or septicemia*—**Adult:** 150-200 mg/kg/day IV in divided doses q 3 or 4 hr; may give IM after 3 days.† **Child:** 100-200 mg/kg IV daily in divided doses q 3 or 4 hr; may give IM after 3 days.†

➤ *Uncomplicated gonorrhea*—**Adult:** 3.5 g PO with 1 g probenecid in 1 dose.†

➤ *Prophylaxis for Salmonella in HIV patient*—**Adult:** 50-100 mg PO qid × several mo.†

➤ *Prophylaxis for bacterial endocarditis before dental or minor respiratory procedures*—**Adult:** 2 g (IV or IM) 30 min before procedure.† **Child:** 50 mg/kg IV or IM 30 min before procedure.†

**ampicillin sodium and
sulbactam sodium**
Unasyn

Aminopenicillin and beta-lactamase inhibitor combination; antibiotic
PRC: B

Available forms
Injection: 1.5, 3 g (1 or 2 g ampicillin sodium and 0.5 or 1 g sulbactam sodium, respectively)

Indications & dosages
➤ *Intra-abdominal, GYN, and skin-structure infection*—**Adult:** 1.5-3 g IM or IV q 6 hr. Max, 4 g sulbactam and 8 g ampicillin (12 g) of combined drugs) daily.†

➤ *Skin-structure infection*—**Child ≥ 1 yr and ≥ 40 kg:** 1.5-3 g IM or IV q 6 hr. Max,

---

§ Adjust in immunocompromised patients　　　　　¶ Adjust in debilitated patients

4 g sulbactam and 8 g ampicillin/d. Max duration, 14 d.† **Child ≥ 1 yr and ≤ 40 kg:** 300 mg/kg/d IV divided equally q 6 hr. Max duration, 14 d.†

amprenavir
Agenerase

HIV protease inhibitor, sulfonamide; anti-retroviral
PRC: C

Available forms
Capsules: 50, 150 mg; *Oral solution:* 15 mg/ml

Indications & dosages
➤ *HIV-1 infection*—**Adult, child 13-16 yr ≥ 50 kg:** *Capsules:* 1,200 mg PO bid.‡ *Oral solution:* 1,400 mg PO bid.†, ‡ **Child 13-16 yr < 50 kg, 4-12 yr:** *Capsules:* 20 mg/kg PO bid or 15 mg/kg PO tid (max, 2,400 mg/d).‡ *Oral solution:* 22.5 mg/kg PO (1.5 ml/kg) bid or 17 mg/ kg PO (1.1 ml/kg) tid (max, 2,800 mg/d). Give with other antiretrovirals.†, ‡

anakinra
Kineret

Lymphokine immunoregulator; immuno-logic drug, antirheumatic
PRC: B

Available forms
Injection: 100 mg/ml in a prefilled glass syringe

Indications & dosages
➤ *Moderately to severely active RA after one or more disease-modifying anti-rheumatics fail*—**Adult:** 100 mg SC daily.

aprepitant
Emend

Substance P and neurokinin-1 receptor antagonist; antiemetic
PRC: B

Available forms
Capsules: 80, 125 mg

Indications & dosages
➤ *With a 5-HT$_3$ antagonist and a cortico-steroid, to prevent acute and delayed nausea and vomiting after highly emeto-genic chemo (including cisplatin)*—**Adult:** 125 mg PO 1 hr before treatment on d 1 of chemo, then 80 mg PO q morning on d 2 and d 3 of chemo.

argatroban
Argatroban

Direct thrombin inhibitor; anticoagulant
PRC: B

Available forms
Injection: 100 mg/ml

Indications & dosages
➤ *Prevention of or therapy for thrombo-sis in patients with heparin-induced thrombocytopenia (HIT)*—**Adult:** 2 mcg/ kg/min, as a continuous IV infusion; ad-just dose until steady-state aPTT is 1.5-3 times initial baseline value, not to ex-

---

ceed 100 sec; max dose, 10 mcg/kg/ min.‡
➤ *Anticoagulation in patients with or at risk for HIT during percutaneous coronary interventions*—**Adult:** 350 mcg/kg IV bolus over 3 to 5 min; continuous IV infusion of 25 mcg/kg/min. Activated clotting time (ACT) should be checked 5-10 min after bolus dose. If ACT < 300 sec, give bolus of 150 mcg/kg and increase infusion to 30 mcg/kg/min; if ACT > 450 sec, decrease infusion to 15 mcg/kg/min. Recheck ACT in 5-10 min. In case of dissection, impending abrupt closure, thrombus formation during procedure, or inability to achieve or maintain ACT > 300 sec, give additional bolus of 150 mcg/kg and increase infusion to 40 mcg/kg/min. Check ACT again after 5-10 min.‡

aripiprazole
Abilify

Psychotropic; atypical antipsychotic
PRC: C

Available forms
Tablets: 5, 10, 15, 20, 30 mg

Indications & dosages
➤ *Schizophrenia*—**Adult:** 10-15 mg PO daily; increase to max daily dose of 30 mg prn after ≥ 2 wk.
Adjust dose if given with CYP 3A4 or CYP 2D6 inhibitors or CYP 3A4 inducers.

aspirin (acetylsalicylic acid)
ASA, Ascriptin, Bayer Timed-Release, Bufferin, Ecotrin

Salicylate; nonopioid analgesic, antipyretic, anti-inflammatory, platelet aggregation inhibitor
PRC: D

Available forms
Chewing gum: 227.5 mg; *Suppository:* 120, 200, 300, 600 mg; *Tablets:* 325, 500 mg; *Tablets (chewable):* 81 mg; *Tablets (controlled-release):* 800 mg; *Tablets (delayed-release, enteric-coated):* 81, 162, 325, 500, 650, 975 mg; *Tablets (timed-release):* 650 mg

Indications & dosages
➤ *RA, other inflammatory conditions*—**Adult:** 2.4-3.6 g PO daily in divided doses. Maintenance, 3.2-6 g PO daily in divided doses.
➤ *Pain, fever*—**Adult, child > 11 yr:** 325-650 mg PO or PR q 4 hr, prn. **Child 2-11 yr:** 10-15 mg/kg PO or PR q 4 hr; max, 60-80 mg/kg/d.
➤ *MI prevention*—**Adult:** 160-325 mg PO daily.

atazanavir sulfate
Reyataz

HIV-1 protease inhibitor; antiretroviral
PRC: B

Available forms
Capsules: 100, 150, 200 mg

---

§ Adjust in immunocompromised patients   ¶ Adjust in debilitated patients

Indications & dosages

➤ *HIV-1 infection (with other antiretrovirals)*—**Adult:** 400 mg PO daily with food.‡ Reduce atazanavir dosage to 300 mg daily if giving with 100 mg ritonavir daily and either 600 mg efavirenz daily or 300 mg tenofovir disoproxil fumarate daily.

atenolol
Apo-Atenolol*, Nu-Atenol*, Tenormin

Beta blocker; antihypertensive, antianginal
PRC: D

Available forms
Injection: 5 mg/10 ml; *Tablets:* 25, 50, 100 mg

Indications & dosages
➤ *HTN*—**Adult:** 50 mg PO daily; increase to 100 mg daily after 7-14 d.†
➤ *Angina pectoris*—**Adult:** 50 mg PO daily; increase to 100 mg daily after 7 d. Max, 200 mg daily.†
➤ *Acute MI*—**Adult:** 5 mg IV over 5 min; repeat 10 min later. After additional 10 min, 50 mg PO; then 50 mg PO in 12 hr. Then, 100 mg PO daily (or 50 mg bid) ≥ 7 d.†

atomoxetine hydrochloride
Strattera

SSRI; ADHD drug
PRC: C

Available forms
Capsules: 10, 18, 25, 40, 60 mg

Indications & dosages
➤ *ADHD*—**Adult, child > 70 kg:** 40 mg PO daily; increase after 3 d to target dose of 80 mg/d,‡ (as a single am dose, or 2 evenly divided doses in the am and late afternoon or early pm). After 2-4 wk, increase to max of 100 mg/d prn.‡ **Child ≤ 70 kg:** 0.5 mg/kg PO daily; increase after 3 d to target dose of 1.2 mg/kg/d (as a single am dose, or 2 evenly divided doses in the am and late afternoon or early pm). Max, 1.4 mg/kg or 100 mg daily, whichever is less.‡

atorvastatin calcium
Lipitor

HMG-CoA reductase inhibitor; antilipemic
PRC: X

Available forms
Tablets: 10, 20, 40, 80 mg

Indications & dosages
➤ *Primary hypercholesterolemia and mixed dyslipidemia*—**Adult:** 10-20 mg PO daily. Patients who require > 45% reduction in LDL cholesterol, start with 40 mg daily. Range, 10-80 mg daily.
➤ *Homozygous familial hypercholesterolemia*—**Adult:** 10-80 mg PO daily.
➤ *Heterozygous familial hypercholesterolemia*—**Child 10-17 yr:** 10 mg PO daily; max, 20 mg/d. Adjust at intervals of ≥ 4 wk.

atropine sulfate

Anticholinergic, belladonna alkaloid; antiarrhythmic, vagolytic
PRC: C

Available forms

Injection: 0.05, 0.1, 0.3, 0.4, 0.5, 0.8, 1 mg/ml; *Tablets:* 0.4 mg

Indications & dosages

➤ *Symptomatic bradycardia, brady-arrhythmia*—**Adult:** 0.5-1 mg IV push; repeat q 3-5 min to max of 2 mg prn. **Child:** 0.01 mg/kg IV; may repeat q 4-6 hr; max, 0.4 mg or 0.3 mg/m².
➤ *Preop, to diminish secretions and block cardiac vagal reflexes*—**Adult, child ≥ 20 kg:** 0.4-0.6 mg IM or SC 30-60 min before anesthesia. **Child < 20 kg:** 0.01 mg/kg IM or SC (max, 0.4 mg) 30-60 min before anesthesia.

azithromycin
Zithromax

Azalide macrolide; antibiotic
PRC: B

Available forms

Injection: 500 mg; *Oral suspension:* 100, 200 mg/5 ml; *Single-dose powder for oral suspension:* 1 g; *Tablets:* 250, 500, 600 mg

Indications & dosages

➤ *Bacterial exacerbation of COPD, community-acquired pneumonia, pharyngitis, tonsillitis, uncomplicated skin and skin-structure infections*—**Adult, child ≥ 16 yr:** 500 mg PO × 1 dose on d 1; then 250 mg daily on d 2-5. Total dose, 1.5 g. Or, for COPD exacerbation, 500 mg PO daily × 3 d.
➤ *Community-acquired pneumonia*—**Child ≥ 6 mo:** 10 mg/kg PO (max, 500 mg) on d 1; then 5 mg/kg (max, 250 mg) on d 2-5.
➤ *Pharyngitis, tonsillitis:* **Child ≥ 2 yr:** 12 mg/kg daily (max, 500 mg) × 5 d.
➤ *OM*—**Child ≥ 6 mo:** 30 mg/kg PO × 1 dose. Or, 10 mg/kg PO (max, 500 mg) in 1 dose; then 5 mg/kg (max, 250 mg) on d 2-5.
➤ *Non-gonococcal urethritis or cervicitis from* Chlamydia trachomatis—**Adult, child ≥ 16 yr:** 1 g PO in 1 dose.
➤ *Gonococcal urethritis or cervicitis*—**Adult, child ≥ 16 yr:** 2 g PO in 1 dose.
➤ *To prevent disseminated MAC in advanced HIV*—**Adult:** 1,200 mg PO q wk alone or with rifabutin.
➤ *Disseminated MAC in advanced HIV*—**Adult:** 600 mg PO daily with ethambutol 15 mg/kg daily.
➤ *Chancroid caused by* Haemophilus ducreyi—**Adult:** 1 g PO × 1 dose.

aztreonam
Azactam

Monobactam; antibiotic
PRC: B

Available forms

Injection: 500-mg, 1-, 2-g vials

---

§ Adjust in immunocompromised patients   ¶ Adjust in debilitated patients

Indications & dosages

➤ *UTI; septicemia; lower respiratory tract, skin and skin-structure, intra-abdominal, surgical, and GYN infection from susceptible gram-neg aerobic organisms; respiratory infection from* Haemophilus influenzae—**Adult:** 500 mg-2 g IV or IM q 8-12 hr. Severe infection, 2 g q 6-8 hr; max, 8 g daily. **Child 9 mo-15 yr:** 30 mg/kg IV q 6-8 hr; max, 120 mg/kg/d.

baclofen
Kemstro, Lioresal, Lioresal Intrathecal

GABA analogue derivative; skeletal muscle relaxant
PRC: C

Available forms

Intrathecal injection: 50, 500, 2,000 mcg/ml; *Tablets:* 10, 20 mg; *Tablets (orally disintegrating):* 10, 20 mg

Indications & dosages

➤ *Spasticity in MS, spinal cord injury*—**Adult:** 5 mg PO tid × 3 d; then 10 mg tid × 3 d, 15 mg tid × 3 d, 20 mg tid × 3 d. Increase prn to max 80 mg daily.
➤ *Severe spasticity*—**Adult:** Test dose is 1 ml of 50-mcg/ml dilution into intrathecal space by barbotage over ≥ 1 min. If poor response, give 2nd test dose (75 mcg/1.5 ml) 24 hr after 1st. If poor response, give final test dose (100 mcg/2 ml) 24 hr later. Patients unresponsive to final test dose shouldn't have implantable pump. Maintenance, double effective test dose and give over 24 hr. If test dose effectiveness maintains ≥ 12 hr, don't double

dose. After 1st 24 hr, increase dose prn by 10-30% daily.

balsalazide disodium
Colazal

GI drug; anti-inflammatory
PRC: B

Available forms

Capsules: 750 mg

Indications & dosages

➤ *Ulcerative colitis*—**Adult:** 2.25 g PO (three 750-mg capsules) tid for total of 6.75 g daily × 8 wk.

basiliximab
Simulect

Monoclonal antibody; immunosuppressant
PRC: B

Available forms

Injection: 20-mg single-dose vials

Indications & dosages

➤ *With other immunosuppressants, to prevent acute kidney rejection after transplant*—**Adult, child ≥ 35 kg:** 20 mg IV ≤ 2 hr before transplant and 20 mg IV 4 d after transplant. **Child < 35 kg:** 10 mg IV ≤ 2 hr before transplant and 10 mg IV 4 d after transplant.

---

beclomethasone dipropionate
QVAR

Glucocorticoid; anti-inflammatory, anti-asthmatic
PRC: C

Available forms
Oral inhalation aerosol: 40, 80 mcg/metered spray

Indications & dosages
➤ *Asthma*—**Adult, child ≥ 12 yr:** 40-80 mcg bid or 40-160 mcg bid (with inhaled corticosteroids). Max, 320 mcg bid. **Child 5-11 yr:** 40 mcg bid; max, 80 mcg bid.

benazepril hydrochloride
Lotensin

ACE inhibitor; antihypertensive
PRC: C (D, 2nd and 3rd trimesters)

Available forms
Tablets: 5, 10, 20, 40 mg

Indications & dosages
➤ *HTN*—**Adult:** For patient not taking diuretics, 10 mg PO daily. Adjust to 20-40 mg daily in 1-2 doses. For patient taking diuretics, 5 mg PO daily.†

benztropine mesylate
Apo-Benztropine*, Cogentin, PMS Benztropine*

Anticholinergic; antiparkinsonian
PRC: C

Available forms
Injection: 1 mg/ml in 2-ml ampule; *Tablets:* 0.5, 1, 2 mg

Indications & dosages
➤ *Drug-induced extrapyramidal disorders (except tardive dyskinesia)*—**Adult:** 1-4 mg PO or IM daily or bid.
➤ *Dystonic reaction*—**Adult:** 1-2 mg IV or IM; then 1-2 mg PO bid.
➤ *Parkinsonism*—**Adult:** 0.5-6 mg PO or IM daily. Initial dose 0.5-1 mg; increase by 0.5 mg q 5-6 d. Max, 6 mg daily.

betamethasone
Betnesol*, Celestone

betamethasone acetate and betamethasone sodium phosphate
Celestone Soluspan

betamethasone sodium phosphate
Celestone Phosphate

Glucocorticoid; anti-inflammatory
PRC: C

Available forms
betamethasone *Syrup:* 600 mcg/5 ml; *Tablets:* 600 mcg; *Tablets (effervescent):* 500 mcg*; **acetate and sodium phos-**

---

§ Adjust in immunocompromised patients　　　　　¶ Adjust in debilitated patients

phate *Injection (suspension):* acetate 3 mg and sodium phosphate (equivalent to 3 mg base)/ml; **sodium phosphate** *Injection:* 4 mg (equivalent to 3-mg base)/ml in 5 ml

Indications & dosages

➤ *Severe inflammation, immunosuppression*—**Adult:** 0.6-7.2 mg PO daily; or 0.5-9 mg IM, IV, or into joint or soft tissue daily. Or, 6-12 mg sodium phosphate-acetate suspension injected into large joints or 1.5-6 mg injected into small joints. Give both injections q 1-2 wk prn. *Note:* Don't give sodium phosphate-acetate suspension mixture IV.

betamethasone dipropionate
Alphatrex, Diprolene, Diprolene AF, Diprosone, Maxivate

betamethasone valerate
Betatrex, Beta-Val, Betnovate*, Luxiq, Valisone

Topical glucocorticoid; anti-inflammatory
PRC: C

Available forms
dipropionate *Aerosol:* 0.1%; *Cream, lotion, ointment:* 0.05%; **valerate** *Cream:* 0.01%, 0.05%, 0.1%; *Foam:* 0.12%; *Lotion, ointment:* 0.1%

Indications & dosages
➤ *Dermatitis*—**Adult, child:** Clean area; apply cream, ointment, lotion, or aerosol sparingly. Give dipropionate daily or bid; give valerate daily to qid.

betaxolol hydrochloride
Betoptic, Betoptic S

Beta blocker; antiglaucoma drug
PRC: C

Available forms
Ophthalmic solution: 0.5%; *Ophthalmic suspension:* 0.25%

Indications & dosages
➤ *Chronic open-angle glaucoma, ocular HTN*—**Adult:** 1 or 2 drops 0.5% solution or 0.25% suspension bid.

bimatoprost
Lumigan

Prostaglandin analogue; antiglaucoma drug, ocular antihypertensive
PRC: C

Available forms
Ophthalmic solution: 0.03%

Indications & dosages
➤ *Reduce IOP in patients with open-angle glaucoma or ocular HTN*—**Adult:** 1 drop in affected eye q pm.

bisacodyl
Bisac-Evac, Bisacodyl Uniserts, Correctol, Dulcolax, Feen-a-mint, Fleet Bisacodyl, Fleet Laxative

Diphenylmethane derivative; stimulant laxative
PRC: NR

Available forms

Suppository: 10 mg; *Tablets (enteric-coated):* 5 mg

Indications & dosages

➤ *Constipation, bowel preparation*—**Adult, child > 12 yr:** 10-15 mg PO in am or pm; max, 30 mg PO or 10 mg PR for evacuation before exam or surgery. **Child 6-12 yr:** 5 mg PO or PR hs or am.

bivalirudin

Angiomax

Direct thrombin inhibitor; anticoagulant
PRC: B

Available forms

Injection: 250-mg vial

Indications & dosages

➤ *Unstable angina in patient undergoing percutaneous transluminal coronary angioplasty (PTCA)*—**Adult:** 1 mg/kg IV bolus just before PTCA; then begin 4-hr IV infusion at 2.5 mg/kg/hr. After the 1st 4-hr infusion, another IV infusion at 0.2 mg/kg/hr ≤ 20 hr may be given prn. Give with 300-325 mg aspirin.†

bortezomib

Velcade

Proteasome inhibitor; antineoplastic
PRC: D

Available forms

Powder for injection: 3.5 mg

Indications & dosages

➤ *Multiple myeloma that still progresses after at least two therapies*—**Adult:** 1.3 mg/m² by IV bolus twice wkly for 2 wk (days 1, 4, 8, and 11) followed by a 10-d rest period (days 12-21). This 3-wk period is 1 treatment cycle. If patient develops a grade 3 nonhematologic or a grade 4 hematologic toxicity (excluding neuropathy), withhold drug; restart at a 25% reduced dose when toxicity has resolved. If patient has neuropathic pain, peripheral neuropathy, or both, adjust dosage.

bosentan

Tracleer

Endothelin receptor antagonist; antihypertensive
PRC: X

Available forms

Tablets: 62.5, 125 mg

Indications & dosages

➤ *To improve WHO class III or IV symptoms of pulmonary arterial HTN*—**Adult:** 62.5 mg PO bid × 4 wk. Increase to maintenance dose of 125 mg PO bid. In patients who develop aminotransferase abnormalities, decrease or stop drug until levels return to normal.

---

§ Adjust in immunocompromised patients   ¶ Adjust in debilitated patients

bromocriptine mesylate
Parlodel

Dopamine receptor agonist, semisynthetic ergot alkaloid, dopaminergic agonist; antiparkinsonian, prolactin release inhibitor, growth hormone release inhibitor
PRC: B

Available forms
Capsules: 5 mg; *Tablets:* 2.5 mg

Indications & dosages
➤ *Amenorrhea, galactorrhea, infertility—* **Woman:** 0.5-2.5 mg PO daily; increase by 2.5 mg daily at 3-7-d intervals prn. Therapeutic dose, 2.5-15 mg/d.
➤ *Parkinson's disease—* **Adult:** 1.25 mg PO bid with meal; increase q 14-28 d. Max, 100 mg daily prn.
➤ *Acromegaly—* **Adult:** 1.25-2.5 mg PO with snack hs × 3 d. Increase by 1.25-2.5 mg q 3-7 d prn. Max, 100 mg/d.

budesonide
Entocort EC

Glucocorticosteroid; anti-inflammatory
PRC: C

Available forms
Capsules: 3 mg

Indications & dosages
➤ *Mild to moderate active Crohn's disease of the ileum or ascending colon—* **Adult:** 9 mg PO once daily in am × ≤ 8 wk. For recurrent episodes, a repeat 8-wk course may be given.‡ May taper to 6 mg PO daily × 2 wk before stopping.

budesonide (nasal)
Rhinocort Aqua

Corticosteroid; anti-inflammatory
PRC: C

Available forms
Nasal spray: 32 mcg/metered spray (7-g canister)

Indications & dosages
➤ *Allergic rhinitis—* **Adult, child ≥ 6 yr:** 2 sprays in each nostril in am and pm, or 4 sprays in each nostril in am.

budesonide (oral inhalant)
Pulmicort Respules, Pulmicort Turbuhaler

Glucocorticosteroid; anti-inflammatory
PRC: B

Available forms
Dry powder inhalation: 200 mcg/dose; *Inhalation suspension:* 0.25 mg/2 ml, 0.5 mg/2 ml

Indications & dosages
➤ *Asthma—* **Adult previously taking bronchodilators only:** 200-400 mcg inhalation bid; max, 400 mcg bid. **Adult previously taking inhalation corticosteroids:** 200-400 mcg inhalation bid; max, 800 mcg bid. **Adult previously taking PO corticosteroids:** 400-800 mcg inhalation bid; max, 800 mcg bid. **Child ≥ 6 yr previously taking bronchodilators only or inhalation corticosteroids:** 200 mcg inhalation bid; max, 400 mcg bid. **Child ≥ 6 yr previously taking PO corticoste-**

roids: Max, 400 mcg bid. **Child 12 mo-8 yr:** (Respules): 0.5-1 mg daily to bid via nebulizer.

bumetanide
Bumex

Loop diuretic; diuretic
PRC: C

Available forms
Injection: 0.25 mg/ml; *Tablets:* 0.5, 1, 2 mg

Indications & dosages
➤ *Edema*—**Adult:** 0.5-2 mg PO daily. May give 2nd or 3rd dose at 4-5 hr intervals prn. Max, 10 mg/d. Or, 0.5-1 mg IV or IM over 1-2 min. May give 2nd or 3rd dose at 2-3 hr intervals prn. Max, 10 mg/d.†

bupropion hydrochloride (antidepressant)
Wellbutrin, Wellbutrin XL, Wellbutrin SR

Aminoketone; antidepressant
PRC: B

Available forms
Tablets (extended-release): 150, 300 mg; *Tablets (immediate-release):* 75, 100 mg; *Tablets (sustained-release):* 100, 150, 200 mg

Indications & dosages
➤ *Depression*—**Adult:** 100 mg immediate-release tablet PO bid × 3 d; then increase to 100 mg tid, prn. If no response after several wk, increase to 150 mg tid. Max, 150 mg/dose. Allow ≥ 6 hr between successive doses. Max, 450 mg/d. Or, 150 mg sustained-release tablet PO q am; increase to 150 mg bid as tolerated as early as d 4 of dosing. Allow ≥ 8 hr between successive doses. Max, 400 mg/d. Or, 150 mg extended-release tablet PO q am; increase to 300 mg daily as tolerated as early as d 4 of dosing. Allow ≥ 24 hr between successive doses. Max, 450 mg/d.†, ‡

bupropion hydrochloride (nicotine replacement)
Zyban

Norepinephrine, serotonin, and dopamine inhibitor; nicotine replacement
PRC: B

Available forms
Tablets (sustained-release): 150 mg

Indications & dosages
➤ *Smoking cessation*—**Adult:** 150 mg PO daily × 3 d; max, 300 mg PO daily in 2 divided doses ≥ 8 hr apart.

buspirone hydrochloride
BuSpar

Azaspirodecanedione derivative; anxiolytic
PRC: B

Available forms
Tablets: 5, 10, 15 mg

Indications & dosages
➤ *Anxiety*—**Adult:** 5 mg PO tid; increase q 3 d in 5-mg increments. Maintenance,

20-30 mg PO daily in divided doses. Max, 60 mg/d.

butorphanol tartrate
Stadol, Stadol NS

Opioid agonist-antagonist, opioid partial agonist; analgesic, adjunct to anesthesia
PRC: C; CSS: IV

Available forms
Injection: 1, 2 mg/ml; *Nasal spray:* 10 mg/ml

Indications & dosages
➤ *Pain*—**Adult:** 1-4 mg IM q 3-4 hr prn or around-the-clock; or 0.5-2 mg IV q 3-4 hr prn or around-the-clock. Max, 4 mg/dose. Or, 1 mg nasally (one spray in each nostril). If no relief in 60-90 min, give 2nd dose. May repeat sequence in 3-4 hr.
➤ *Preop anesthesia or preanesthesia*—**Adult:** 2 mg IM 60-90 min preop.

calcitonin (salmon)
Miacalcin, Salmonine

Thyroid hormone; hypocalcemic
PRC: C

Available forms
Injection: 200 IU/ml, 2-ml ampule; *Nasal spray:* 200 IU/activation in 2-ml bottle

Indications & dosages
➤ *Paget's disease*—**Adult:** 100 IU daily SC or IM; maintenance, 50 IU daily or 50-100 IU 3 times/wk.
➤ *Hypercalcemia*—**Adult:** 4 IU/kg q 12 hr IM. If poor response after 1 or 2 d, give

8 IU/kg IM q 12 hr. If poor response after ≥ 2 d, increase to max 8 IU/kg IM q 6 hr.
➤ *Osteoporosis*—**Adult:** 100 IU daily IM or SC. Or, 200 IU (1 spray) daily intranasally, alternating nostrils daily.

calcitriol (1,25-dihydroxycholecalciferol)
Calcijex, Rocaltrol

Vitamin D analogue; antihypocalcemic
PRC: A (D, doses > RDA)

Available forms
Capsules: 0.25, 0.5 mcg; *Injection:* 1, 2 mcg/ml; *Oral solution:* 1 mcg/ml

Indications & dosages
➤ *Hypocalcemia in long-term dialysis*—**Adult:** 0.25 mcg PO daily. Increase by 0.25 mcg daily q 4-8 wk. Maintenance, 0.25 mcg every other d; max 1.25 mcg daily.
➤ *Hypoparathyroidism, pseudohypoparathyroidism*—**Adult, child > 6 yr:** 0.25 mcg PO daily. Increase at 2-4 wk intervals prn. Maintenance, 0.5-2 mcg daily.
➤ *Hypoparathyroidism*—**Child 1-5 yr:** 0.25-0.75 mcg PO daily.

calcium carbonate
Alka-Mints, Calci-Chew, Chooz, Os-Cal 500, Tums 500

Calcium supplement; electrolyte balance drug
PRC: NR

Available forms

Contains 400 mg or 20 mEq elemental calcium/g. *Capsules:* 1,250 mg; *Gum:* 300, 450, 500 mg; *Oral suspension:* 1,250 mg/5 ml; *Powder packet:* 6.5 g (2,400 mg calcium)/packet; *Tablets:* 500, 600, 650, 667, 1,250, 1,500 mg; *Tablets (chewable):* 350, 420, 500, 750, 850, 1,000, 1,250 mg

Indications & dosages

➤ *Antacid*—**Adult:** 350 mg-1.5 g PO or 2 pieces of chewing gum 1 hr pc and hs prn.
➤ *Dietary supplement*—**Adult:** 500 mg-2 g PO bid-qid.

> ### calcium salts
> Calciject* (chloride), Calphron (acetate), Citracal (citrate), Neo-Calglucon (glubionate), PhosLo (acetate), Posture (phosphate)

Calcium supplement; electrolyte balance drug, cardiotonic
PRC: C

Available forms

acetate (253 mg or 12.7 mEq elemental calcium/g) *Capsules:* 333.5, 667 mg; *Gelcaps:* 667 mg; *Injection:* 0.5 mEq elemental calcium/ml; *Tablets:* 667 mg; **chloride** (270 mg or 13.7 mEq elemental calcium/g) *Injection:* 10% solution in 10-ml ampule, vial, syringe; **citrate** (211 mg or 10.6 mEq elemental calcium/g) *Tablets:* 950 mg, 1.04 g; *Tablets (effervescent):* 2.376 g; **glubionate** (64 mg or 3.2 mEq elemental calcium/g) *Syrup:* 1.8 g/5 ml; **gluceptate** (82 mg or 4.1 mEq elemental

calcium/g) *Injection:* 1.1g/5 ml in 5-ml ampule, 10-ml vial; **gluconate** (90 mg or 4.5 mEq elemental calcium/g) *Injection:* 10% solution in 10-ml ampule, 10-, 50-ml vials; *Tablets:* 500, 650 mg, 1 g; **lactate** (130 mg or 6.5 mEq elemental calcium/g) *Tablets:* 325, 650 mg; **phosphate, tribasic** (400 mg or 20 mEq elemental calcium/g) *Tablets:* 1,565 mg

Indications & dosages

➤ *Hypocalcemic emergency*—**Adult:** 7-14 mEq IV (as 10% gluconate solution, 2-10% chloride solution, or 22% gluceptate solution). **Child:** 1-7 mEq IV. **Infant:** Up to 1 mEq IV.
➤ *Hypocalcemic tetany*—**Adult:** 4.5-16 mEq IV. Repeat prn. **Child:** 0.5-0.7 mEq/kg IV tid or qid until controlled. **Neonate:** 2.4 mEq/kg IV daily in divided doses.
➤ *Cardiac arrest*—**Adult:** 0.027-0.054 mEq/kg chloride IV, 4.5-6.3 mEq gluceptate IV, or 2.3-3.7 mEq gluconate IV. **Child:** 0.27 mEq/kg IV. Repeat in 10 min prn; check calcium level before giving further doses.
➤ *Magnesium intoxication*—**Adult:** 7 mEq IV. Give subsequent doses prn.
➤ *Exchange transfusion*—**Adult:** 1.35 mEq IV with each 100 ml citrated blood. **Neonate:** 0.45 mEq IV after each 100 ml citrated blood.
➤ *Hyperphosphatemia*—**Adult:** 1,334-2,000 mg PO acetate tid with meals. Dialysis patient needs 3-4 tablets with meals.

---

§ Adjust in immunocompromised patients ¶ Adjust in debilitated patients

candesartan cilexetil
Atacand

Selective angiotensin II receptor antagonist; antihypertensive
PRC: C (D, 2nd and 3rd trimesters)

Available forms
Tablets: 4, 8, 16, 32 mg

Indications & dosages
➤ *HTN*—**Adult:** 16 mg PO daily as monotherapy; range, 8-32 mg PO once daily or divided bid.

captopril
Apo-Capto*, Capoten, Novo-Captopril*

ACE inhibitor; antihypertensive, adjunct therapy for HF
PRC: C (D, 2nd and 3rd trimesters)

Available forms
Tablets: 12.5, 25, 50, 100 mg

Indications & dosages
➤ *HTN*—**Adult:** 25 mg PO bid or tid. In 1-2 wk, increase to 50 mg bid or tid prn. If BP is uncontrolled after another 1-2 wk, add diuretic. If further BP reduction is needed, increase to 150 mg tid with diuretic. Max, 450 mg daily.
➤ *HF, reduce HF after MI*—**Adult:** 6.25-12.5 mg PO tid. Increase to 50 mg tid prn. Max, 450 mg daily.

carbamazepine
Apo-Carbamazepine*, Carbatrol, Epitol, Novo-Carbamaz*, Tegretol, Tegretol-XR

Iminostilbene derivative; anticonvulsant, analgesic
PRC: D

Available forms
Capsules (extended-release): 200, 300 mg; *Oral suspension:* 100 mg/5 ml; *Tablets:* 200 mg; *Tablets (chewable):* 100 mg; *Tablets (extended-release):* 100, 200, 400 mg

Indications & dosages
➤ *Seizures*—**Adult, child > 12 yr:** 200 mg tablet PO bid or 100 mg suspension PO qid. Increase each wk by 200 mg daily, in divided doses at 6-8 hr intervals prn. Max, 1 g/d in child 12-15 yr or 1.2 g/d in child > 15 yr. **Child 6-12 yr:** 100-mg tablet PO bid or 50 mg suspension PO qid. Increase each wk by 100 mg PO daily. Max, 1 g/d. **Child < 6 yr:** 10-20 mg/kg/d PO bid or tid (tablets) or qid (suspension). Max, 35 mg/kg/d.

carvedilol
Coreg

Beta blocker; vasodilator, antihypertensive
PRC: C

Available forms
Tablets: 3.125, 6.25, 12.5, 25 mg

Indications & dosages
➤ *HTN*—**Adult:** 6.25 mg PO bid. Take standing BP 1 hr after initial dose. If toler-

---

ated, continue dose × 7-14 d. Increase to 12.5 mg PO bid × 7-14 d prn, monitoring BP. Max, 25 mg PO bid. Reduce dose in patients with pulse rate < 55 beats/min.
➤ *HF*—**Adult:** 3.125 mg PO bid × 2 wk; if tolerated, increase to 6.25 mg PO bid. May double dose q 2 wk. Max for patients ≤ 85 kg, 25 mg PO bid; patients > 85 kg, 50 mg PO bid. Reduce dose in patients with pulse rate < 55 beats/min.
➤ *Left ventricular dysfunction post-MI*—**Adult:** Initially 6.25 mg PO bid × 3-10 d; then 12.5 mg bid up to 25 mg bid.

caspofungin acetate
Cancidas

Glucan synthesis inhibitor; antifungal
PRC: C

Available forms
Lyophilized powder for injection: 50-, 70-mg single-use vials

Indications & dosages
➤ *Invasive aspergillosis in patients refractory to or intolerant of other therapy*—**Adult:** Single 70-mg loading dose on d 1, followed by 50 mg daily thereafter. Give by slow IV infusion over about 1 hr. Treatment length based on severity of underlying disease, recovery from immunosuppression, and patient response.†

cefaclor
Ceclor

2nd-generation cephalosporin; antibiotic
PRC: B

Available forms
Capsules: 250, 500 mg; *Oral suspension:* 125, 187, 250, 375 mg/5 ml; *Tablets (extended-release):* 375, 500 mg

Indications & dosages
➤ *UTI; respiratory, skin, soft-tissue infection; OM*—**Adult:** 250-500 mg PO q 8 hr. For adult with pharyngitis or OM, may give daily dose in 2 equally divided doses q 12 hr. **Child:** 20 mg/kg daily PO in divided doses q 8 hr. More serious infection, 40 mg/kg daily; max 1 g daily. For child with pharyngitis or OM, may give daily dose in 2 equally divided doses q 12 hr.

cefadroxil monohydrate
Duricef

1st-generation cephalosporin; antibiotic
PRC: B

Available forms
Capsules: 500 mg; *Oral suspension:* 125, 250, 500 mg/5 ml; *Tablets:* 1 g

Indications & dosages
➤ *UTI; skin, soft-tissue infection; pharyngitis; tonsillitis*—**Adult:** 1-2 g PO daily, given daily or bid. **Child:** 30 mg/kg PO daily in 2 divided doses q 12 hr.†

---

§ Adjust in immunocompromised patients　　　　¶ Adjust in debilitated patients

cefazolin sodium
Ancef

1st-generation cephalosporin; antibiotic
PRC: B

Available forms
Infusion: 500 mg, 1 g/50-ml vial; *Injection (parenteral):* 500 mg, 1 g

Indications & dosages
➤ *Prophylaxis in contaminated surgery*—**Adult:** 1 g IM or IV 30-60 min preop; then 0.5-1 g IM or IV q 6-8 hr × 24 hr. For surgery > 2 hr, may give another 0.5-1 g IM intraop. Therapy may continue × 3-5 d prn.†
➤ *Respiratory, biliary, GU, skin, soft-tissue, bone, joint infection; septicemia; endocarditis*—**Adult:** 250 mg IM or IV q 8 hr to 1.5 g PO q 6 hr. Max, 12 g/d. **Infant > 1 mo:** 25-50 mg/kg or 1.25 g/m^2 daily IM or IV in 3 or 4 divided doses. May increase to 100 mg/kg/d.†

cefdinir
Omnicef

3rd-generation cephalosporin; antibiotic
PRC: B

Available forms
Capsules: 300 mg; *Suspension:* 125 mg/5 ml

Indications & dosages
➤ *Community-acquired pneumonia, exacerbation of chronic bronchitis, maxillary sinusitis, OM, uncomplicated skin and skin-structure infection*—**Adult, child ≥ 13 yr:** 300 mg PO q 12 hr or 600 mg PO q 24 hr × 10 d. (Use q-12-hr doses for pneumonia and skin infection.) **Child 6 mo-12 yr:** 7 mg/kg PO q 12 hr or 14 mg/kg PO q 24 hr × 10 d; max 600 mg daily. (Use q-12-hr doses for skin infection.)†
➤ *Pharyngitis, tonsillitis*—**Adult, child ≥ 13 yr:** 300 mg PO q 12 hr × 5-10 d or 600 mg PO q 24 hr × 10 d. **Child 6 mo-12 yr:** 7 mg/kg PO q 12 hr × 5-10 d or 14 mg/kg PO q 24 hr × 10 d.†

cefditoren pivoxil
Spectracef

Semisynthetic 3rd-generation cephalosporin; antibiotic
PRC: B

Available forms
Tablets: 200 mg

Indications & dosages
➤ *Acute bacterial exacerbation of chronic bronchitis from* Haemophilus influenzae, H. parainfluenzae, Streptococcus pneumoniae, Moraxella catarrhalis—**Adult, child ≥ 12 yr:** 400 mg PO bid with meals × 10 d.†
➤ *Pharyngitis or tonsillitis from* Streptococcus pyogenes—**Adult, child ≥ 2 yr:** 200 mg PO bid with meals × 10 d.†
➤ *Uncomplicated skin and skin-structure infection from* S. pyogenes—**Adult, child ≥ 12 yr:** 200 mg PO bid with meals ×10 d.†

---

cefepime hydrochloride
Maxipime

Semisynthetic 4th-generation cephalosporin; antibiotic
PRC: B

Available forms
Injection: 500 mg; 1, 2 g

Indications & dosages
➤ *UTI*—**Adult, child ≥ 12 yr:** 0.5-1 g (IM for *Escherichia coli* infection) or IV over 30 min q 12 hr × 7-10 d.†
➤ *UTI, pyelonephritis, skin infection, pneumonia, febrile neutropenic pediatric patients*—**Child 2 mo-16 yr ≤ 40 kg:** 50 mg/kg/dose IV over 30 min q 12 hr (q 8 hr in febrile neutropenia) × 7-10 d; max 2 g/dose.†
➤ *Severe UTI*—**Adult, child ≥ 12 yr:** 2 g IV over 30 min q 12 hr × 10 d.†
➤ *Pneumonia*—**Adult, child ≥ 12 yr:** 1-2 g IV over 30 min q 12 hr × 10 d.†

cefoperazone sodium
Cefobid

3rd-generation cephalosporin; antibiotic
PRC: B

Available forms
Injection: 1, 2 g

Indications & dosages
➤ *Respiratory, intra-abdominal, GYN, skin infection; bacteremia; septicemia*—**Adult:** 1-2 g q 12 hr IM or IV. Severe infections may require up to 12 g daily divided q 6-12 hr.‡

cefotaxime sodium
Claforan

3rd-generation cephalosporin; antibiotic
PRC: B

Available forms
Infusion: 1, 2 g; *Injection:* 500 mg; 1, 2 g

Indications & dosages
➤ *Periop prophylaxis in contaminated surgery*—**Adult, child ≥ 50 kg:** 1 g IM or IV 30-90 min preop. For cesarean section, 1 g IM or IV when umbilical cord is clamped; then 1 g IM or IV 6 and 12 hr later.†
➤ *UTI; lower respiratory tract, CNS, skin, bone, joint infection; GYN, intra-abdominal infection; bacteremia; septicemia*—**Adult:** 1 g IV or IM q 6-8 hr. Max, 12 g daily. **Child 1 mo-12 yr or < 50 kg:** 50-180 mg/kg/d IM or IV in 4-6 divided doses. **Neonate ≤ 1 wk:** 50 mg/kg IV q 12hr. **Neonate 1-4 wk:** 50 mg/kg IV q 8 hr.†

cefotetan disodium
Cefotan

2nd-generation cephalosporin, cephamycin; antibiotic
PRC: B

Available forms
Infusion: 1, 2 g piggyback; *Injection:* 1, 2 g

Indications & dosages
➤ *UTI; lower respiratory tract, GYN, skin, skin-structure, intra-abdominal, bone,*

§ Adjust in immunocompromised patients ¶ Adjust in debilitated patients

joint infection—**Adult:** 1-2 g IV or IM q 12 hr × 5-10 d. Max 6 g/d.†
➤ *Periop prophylaxis*—**Adult:** 1-2 g IV × 1 dose 30-60 min preop. In cesarean section, give dose when umbilical cord is clamped.†

cefoxitin sodium
Mefoxin

2nd-generation cephalosporin, cephamycin; antibiotic
PRC: B

Available forms
Injection: 1, 2 g

Indications & dosages
➤ *Respiratory, GU tract, skin, soft-tissue, bone, joint, bloodstream, intra-abdominal infection; periop prophylaxis*—**Adult:** 1-2 g IV q 6-8 hr; max 12 g/d. **Child ≥ 3 mo:** 80-160 mg/kg/d IV in 4-6 equally divided doses; max 12 g/d.†
➤ *Surgery prophylaxis*—**Adult:** 2 g IM or IV 30-60 min preop; then 2 g IM or IV q 6 hr × 24 hr (72 hr after prosthetic arthroplasty). **Child ≥ 3 mo:** 30-40 mg/kg IM or IV 30-60 min preop; then 30-40 mg/kg q 6 hr × 24 hr (72 hr after prosthetic arthroplasty).†
➤ *Acute PID*—**Adult:** 2 g IV q 6 hr with 100 mg doxycycline IV or PO q 12 hr for at least 2 d after improvement; doxycycline should be continued to complete total of 14 d. Or, 2 g IM × 1 dose with 1 g probenecid, followed by 100 mg doxycycline PO bid × 14 d.†

cefpodoxime proxetil
Vantin

3rd-generation cephalosporin; antibiotic
PRC: B

Available forms
Oral suspension: 50, 100 mg/5 ml in 100-ml bottles; *Tablets (film-coated):* 100, 200 mg

Indications & dosages
➤ *Community-acquired pneumonia*—**Adult, child ≥ 13 yr:** 200 mg PO q 12 hr × 14 d.†
➤ *Exacerbation of chronic bronchitis*—**Adult, child ≥ 13 yr:** 200 mg PO q 12 hr × 10 d.†
➤ *Sinusitis from* Haemophilus influenzae, Streptococcus pneumoniae, *or* Moraxella catarrhalis—**Adult, child ≥ 12 yr:** 200 mg PO q 12 hr × 10 d. **Child 2 mo-11 yr:** 5 mg/kg PO q 12 hr × 10 d; max 200 mg/dose.†
➤ *UTI from* Escherichia coli, Klebsiella pneumoniae, Proteus mirabilis, *or* Staphylococcus saprophyticus—**Adult:** 100 mg PO q 12 hr × 7 d.†

cefprozil
Cefzil

2nd-generation cephalosporin; antibiotic
PRC: B

Available forms
Oral suspension: 125, 250 mg/5 ml; *Tablets:* 250, 500 mg

Indications & dosages

➤ *Pharyngitis or tonsillitis from* Staphylococcus pyogenes—**Adult, child ≥ 13 yr:** 500 mg PO daily × 10 d.† **Child 2-12 yr:** 7.5 mg/kg PO q 12 hr × 10 d.†
➤ *OM from* Streptococcus pneumoniae, Haemophilus influenzae, *or* Moraxella catarrhalis—**Infant, child 6 mo-12 yr:** 15 g/kg PO q 12 hr × 10 d.†
➤ *Acute sinusitis*—**Adult, child ≥ 13 yr:** 250-500 mg PO q 12 hr ×10 d. **Child 6 mo-12 yr:** 7.5-15 mg/kg PO q 12 hr × 10 d.†

ceftazidime
Ceptaz, Fortaz, Tazicef, Tazidime

3rd-generation cephalosporin; antibiotic
PRC: B

Available forms
Injection (with arginine): 1, 2 g; *Injection (with sodium carbonate):* 500 mg; 1, 2 g

Indications & dosages
➤ *UTI; lower respiratory tract, GYN, intra-abdominal, CNS, skin infection; bacteremia; septicemia*—**Adult, child ≥ 12 yr:** 1 g IV or IM q 8-12 hr; max 6 g daily.† **Child 1 mo-12 yr:** 30-50 mg/kg IV q 8 hr (sodium carbonate prep).† **Neonate ≤ 4 wk:** 30 mg/kg IV q 12 hr (sodium carbonate prep).†

ceftizoxime sodium
Cefizox

3rd-generation cephalosporin; antibiotic
PRC: B

Available forms
Injection: 500 mg; 1, 2 g

Indications & dosages
➤ *UTI; lower respiratory tract, GYN, intra-abdominal, bone, joint, skin infection; bacteremia; septicemia; meningitis*—**Adult:** 1-2 g IV or IM q 8-12 hr; max, 2 g q 4 hr. **Child > 6 mo:** 33-50 mg/kg IV q 6-8 hr, up to 200 mg/kg/d in divided doses. Max, 12 g/d.†

ceftriaxone sodium
Rocephin

3rd-generation cephalosporin; antibiotic
PRC: B

Available forms
Injection: 250, 500 mg; 1, 2 g

Indications & dosages
➤ *Infection*—**Adult:** 1-2 g IM or IV daily or bid.
➤ *Serious infection of lower respiratory or urinary tract; GYN, bone, joint, intra-abdominal, skin infection; bacteremia; septicemia; Lyme disease*—**Adult, child > 12 yr:** 1-2 g IM or IV daily or in equally divided doses bid; max, 4 g/d. **Child ≤ 12 yr:** 50-75 mg/kg IM or IV; max, 2 g/d in divided doses q 12 hr.
➤ *Meningitis*—**Adult, child:** 100 mg/kg IM or IV (max, 4 g); then 100 mg/kg/d IM

or IV given daily or in divided doses q 12 hr. Max, 4 g/d × 7-14 d.

cefuroxime axetil
Ceftin

cefuroxime sodium
Zinacef

2nd-generation cephalosporin; antibiotic
PRC: B

Available forms
axetil *Suspension:* 125, 250 mg/5 ml; *Tablets:* 125, 250, 500 mg; **sodium** *Infusion:* 750 mg; 1.5 g premixed, frozen solution; *Injection:* 750 mg; 1.5 g

Indications & dosages
➤ *Serious infection; periop prophylaxis (injection); OM, pharyngitis; tonsillitis; UTI; lower respiratory tract, skin, skin-structure infection (PO)*—**Adult, child ≥ 12 yr:** 750 mg-1.5 g sodium IM or IV q 8 hr × 5-10 d; 1.5 g IM or IV q 6 hr in certain situations. **Child, infant > 3 mo:** 50-100 mg/kg/d sodium IM or IV in divided doses q 6-8 hr.†
➤ *Bacterial meningitis*—**Adult, child ≥ 12 yr:** Up to 3 g IV q 8 hr. Or, 250-500 mg axetil PO q 12 hr. **Child, infant > 3 mo:** 200-240 mg/kg IV in divided doses q 6-8 hr. Or, 125 mg axetil PO q 12 hr.†
➤ *OM*—**Child < 2 yr:** 125 mg PO q 12 hr. **Child ≥ 2 yr:** 250 mg PO q 12 hr.†
➤ *Early Lyme disease from* Borrelia burgdorferi—**Adult, child ≥ 13 yr:** 500 mg PO bid × 20 d.†
➤ *Sinusitis*—**Adult, child ≥ 13 yr:** 250 mg tablet PO bid × 10 d. **Child 3 mo-**

12 yr: 30 mg/kg suspension PO daily in 2 divided doses × 10 d. Max suspension dose, 1,000 mg/d. Or, 250 mg tablet PO bid × 10 d.

celecoxib
Celebrex

COX-2 inhibitor; NSAID
PRC: C

Available forms
Capsules: 100, 200, 400 mg

Indications & dosages
➤ *Familial adenomatous polyposis*—**Adult:** 400 mg PO bid with food ≤ 6 mo.‡
➤ *OA*—**Adult:** 200 mg PO once daily or divided equally bid. In patients < 50 kg, start at lowest dose.‡
➤ *RA*—**Adult:** 100-200 mg PO bid. In patients < 50 kg, start at lowest dose.‡
➤ *Acute pain, primary dysmenorrhea*—**Adult:** Initially 400 mg PO; follow with 200-mg dose if needed on the 1st d. On subsequent d, 200 mg PO bid prn.

cephalexin hydrochloride
Keftab

cephalexin monohydrate
Apo-Cephalex*, Biocef, Keflex

1st-generation cephalosporin; antibiotic
PRC: B

Available forms
hydrochloride *Tablets:* 500 mg; **monohydrate** *Capsules:* 250, 500 mg; *Oral sus-*

pension: 125, 250 mg/5 ml; *Tablets:* 250, 500 mg; 1 g

Indications & dosages
➤ *Respiratory, GI tract, skin, soft-tissue, bone, joint infection; OM from* Escherichia coli *and other coliform bacteria, group A beta-hemolytic strep,* Klebsiella, Proteus mirabilis, Streptococcus pneumoniae, *and staph*—**Adult:** 250 mg-1 g PO q 6 hr. **Child:** 6-12 mg/kg monohydrate PO q 6 hr. Max, 25 mg/kg q 6 hr.

cetirizine hydrochloride
Zyrtec

Selective H$_1$-receptor antagonist; antihistamine
PRC: B

Available forms
Oral solution: 5 mg/5 ml; *Tablets:* 5, 10 mg

Indications & dosages
➤ *Seasonal allergic rhinitis*—**Adult, child ≥ 6 yr:** 5 or 10 mg PO daily.‡, † **Child 2-5 yr:** 2.5 mg PO daily. Max, 5 mg/d.‡, †
➤ *Perennial allergic rhinitis, chronic urticaria*—**Adult, child ≥ 6 yr:** 5 or 10 mg PO daily.‡, † **Child 6 mo-5 yr:** 2.5 mg PO daily. **Child 1-5 yr:** 2.5 mg PO daily to max of 2.5 mg PO bid.‡, †

chlordiazepoxide
Libritabs

chlordiazepoxide hydrochloride
Librium, Novo-Poxide*

Benzodiazepine; anxiolytic, anticonvulsant, sedative-hypnotic
PRC: D; CSS: IV

Available forms
chlordiazepoxide *Tablets:* 10, 25 mg; **hydrochloride** *Capsules:* 5, 10, 25 mg; *Powder for injection:* 100-mg ampule

Indications & dosages
➤ *Anxiety*—**Adult:** 5-10 mg PO tid or qid. **Child > 6 yr:** 5 mg PO bid-qid. Max, 10 mg PO bid or tid.
➤ *Severe anxiety*—**Adult:** 20-25 mg PO tid or qid. **Elderly:** 5 mg PO bid-qid.
➤ *Acute alcohol withdrawal*—**Adult:** 50-100 mg PO, IM, or IV; repeat in 2-4 hr prn. Max, 300 mg daily.

cholestyramine
LoCHOLEST, LoCHOLEST Light, Prevalite, Questran, Questran Light

Anion exchange resin; antilipemic, bile acid sequestrant
PRC: B

Available forms
Powder: 378-g cans; 5-, 5.5-, 5.7-, 6.4-, 9-g single-dose packet (1 scoop powder or single-dose packet has 4 g cholestyramine resin)

§ Adjust in immunocompromised patients   ¶ Adjust in debilitated patients

Indications & dosages

➤ *Primary hyperlipidemia or pruritus from partial bile obstruction; primary hypercholesterolemia*—**Adult:** 4 g daily or bid. Maintenance, 8-16 g daily divided into 2 doses. Max, 24 g daily.

cidofovir
Vistide

Nucleotide analogue; antiviral
PRC: C

Available forms
Injection: 75 mg/ml in 5-ml vial

Indications & dosages

➤ *CMV retinitis in AIDS patients*—**Adult:** 5 mg/kg IV over 1 hr in 1 dose/wk × 2 consecutive wk; then maintenance dose, 5 mg/kg IV over 1 hr q 2 wk. Must give probenecid and prehydration with NSS IV at the same time.†

cilostazol
Pletal

Quinolinone phosphodiesterase inhibitor; platelet aggregation inhibitor, vasodilator
PRC: C

Available forms
Tablets: 50, 100 mg

Indications & dosages

➤ *Intermittent claudication*—**Adult:** 100 mg PO bid ≥ 30 min ac or 2 hr pc (am and pm). Decrease to 50 mg PO bid if giving with drug that increases cilostazol levels.

cimetidine
Tagamet, Tagamet HB

H_2*-receptor antagonist; antiulcerative*
PRC: B

Available forms
Injection: 300 mg/2 ml, 300 mg in 50 ml NSS; *Oral liq:* 300 mg/5 ml; *Tablets:* 100, 200, 300, 400, 800 mg

Indications & dosages

➤ *Duodenal ulcer*—**Adult, child > 16 yr:** 800 mg PO hs. Or, 400 mg PO bid or 300 mg qid with meals and hs. Maintenance, 400 mg hs.†
➤ *Hospitalized patients who can't take oral drugs or patients with intractable ulcers or hypersecretory conditions; GI bleeding; to control gastric pH in critically ill patients*—**Adult:** 300 mg dilution in 20 ml by IV push over > 5 min q 6 hr; or, 300 mg dilution in 50 ml IV solution over 15-20 min q 6 hr; or, 300 mg IM q 6 hr (no dilution needed). Max, 2,400 mg daily prn. Or, 900 mg/d (37.5 mg/hr) IV dilution in 100-1,000 ml by continuous IV infusion.†
➤ *Gastric ulcer*—**Adult:** 800 mg PO hs, or 300 mg PO qid × ≤ 8 wk.†
➤ *GERD*—**Adult:** 800 mg PO bid or 400 mg qid ac and hs × 12 wk.†

---

ciprofloxacin
Cipro, Cipro I.V., Cipro XR

Fluoroquinolone; antibiotic
PRC: C

Available forms
Infusion (premixed): 200 mg in 100 ml D₅W, 400 mg in 200 ml D₅W; *Injection:* 200, 400 mg; *Oral suspension:* 250, 500 mg/5 ml (after reconstitution); *Tablets (extended-release, film-coated):* 500 mg; *Tablets (film-coated):* 100, 250, 500, 750 mg

Indications & dosages
➤ *Uncomplicated UTI*—**Adult:** 250 mg PO or 200 mg IV q 12 hr.† Or, 500 mg extended-release PO daily × 3 d.
➤ *Severe UTI; mild to moderate bone, joint, skin, skin-structure infection*—**Adult:** 500 mg PO × 7-14 d (≥ 4-6 wk for bone or joint infection) or 400 mg IV q 12 hr.†
➤ *Complicated UTI caused by* E. coli, Klebsiella pneumoniae, Proteus mirabilis, Enterococcus faecalis, P. aeruginosa; *acute uncomplicated pyelonephritis caused by* E. coli—**Adult:** 1,000 mg (extended-release) PO daily × 7-14 d.†
➤ *Chronic prostatitis from* Escherichia coli *or* Proteus mirabilis—**Adult:** 500 mg PO q 12 hr × 28 d; or, 400 mg IV over 60 min q 12 hr.†
➤ *Sinusitis*—**Adult:** 400 mg IV over 60 min q 12 hr, or 500 mg PO q 12 hr × 10 d.†
➤ *Inhalation anthrax (postexposure)*—**Adult:** 400 mg q 12 hr IV until susceptibility tests are known; then 500 mg PO bid.
Child: 10 mg/kg q 12 hr IV; then 15 mg/kg PO q 12 hr. Max, 800 mg/d IV or 1,000 mg/d PO. **All patients:** Give with 1 or 2 additional antimicrobials. Switch to PO treatment ASAP. Total therapy should last × 60 d.

ciprofloxacin hydrochloride
Ciloxan

Fluoroquinolone; antibiotic
PRC: C

Available forms
Ophthalmic solution: 0.3% (base) in 2.5- and 5-ml containers

Indications & dosages
➤ *Corneal ulcers*—**Adult, child > 12 yr:** 2 drops in affected eye q 15 min × 1st hr; then 2 drops q 30 min for rest of d 1. Give 2 drops q hr on d 2. On d 3-14, 2 drops q 4 hr.
➤ *Conjunctivitis*—**Adult, child > 12 yr:** 1 or 2 drops in affected eye q 2 hr while awake × 1st 2 d. Then 1 or 2 drops q 4 hr while awake × 5 d.

cisplatin (cisplatinum, CDDP)
Platinol, Platinol-AQ

Alkylating agent; antineoplastic
PRC: D

Available forms
Injection: 0.5*, 1 mg/ml

---

§ Adjust in immunocompromised patients   ¶ Adjust in debilitated patients

Indications & dosages

➤ *Metastatic testicular CA*—**Adult:** 20 mg/m^2 IV daily × 5 d. Repeat q 3 wk × 3 cycles or longer.

➤ *Metastatic ovarian CA*—**Adult:** 100 mg/m^2 IV; repeat q 4 wk. Or, 75-100 mg/m^2 IV q 4 wk with cyclophosphamide.

➤ *Bladder CA*—**Adult:** 50-70 mg/m^2 IV q 3-4 wk. In patients with previous antineoplastic or radiation treatment, 50 mg/m^2 q 4 wk.

citalopram hydrobromide
Celexa

SSRI; antidepressant
PRC: C

Available forms
Oral solution: 10 mg/5 ml; *Tablets:* 10, 20, 40 mg

Indications & dosages
➤ *Depression*—**Adult:** 20 mg PO daily, increasing to 40 mg daily after 1 wk. Max, 40 mg/d. Adjust dose in elderly.‡

clarithromycin
Biaxin, Biaxin XL

Macrolide; antibiotic
PRC: C

Available forms
Suspension: 125, 250 mg/5 ml; *Tablets (extended-release):* 500 mg, 14-tablet blister pack; *Tablets (film-coated):* 250, 500 mg

Indications & dosages

➤ *Pharyngitis, tonsillitis from* Streptococcus pyogenes—**Adult:** 250 mg PO q 12 hr × 10 d.† **Child:** 15 mg/kg/d PO in divided doses q 12 hr × 10 d.†

➤ *Maxillary sinusitis from* Streptococcus pneumoniae, Haemophilus influenzae, *or* Moraxella catarrhalis—**Adult:** 500 mg PO q 12 hr × 14 d or 2 extended-release tablets q 24 hr × 14 d.† **Child:** 15 mg/kg/d PO in divided doses q 12 hr × 10 d.†

➤ *MAC disease in HIV infection*—**Adult:** 500 mg PO q 12 hr.† **Child:** 7.5 mg/kg PO (max, 500 mg) q 12 hr.† Adult, child should take with other antimycobacterials for life.

➤ *Helicobacter pylori infection*—**Adult:** Triple-therapy, 500 mg Biaxin with 30 mg lansoprazole and 1 g amoxicillin, all given q 12 hr × 10-14 d or 500 mg Biaxin with 20 mg omeprazole and 1 g amoxicillin, all given q 12 hr × 10 d. Or, Biaxin 500 mg with rabeprazole 20 mg and amoxicillin 1,000 mg all PO bid × 7 d. Or, dual therapy with 500 mg Biaxin q 8 hr and 40 mg omeprazole daily × 14 d.† **Child:** 15 mg/kg/d divided q 12 hr × 10 d.†

➤ *Community-acquired pneumonia from* Chlamydia pneumoniae, Mycoplasma pneumoniae, Streptococcus pneumoniae, Haemophilus influenzae, Haemophilus parainfluenzae, *or* Moraxella catarrhalis—**Adult:** 250 mg PO q 12 hr × 7-14 d (for Haemophilus influenzae, duration of therapy is 7 d). Don't use conventional tablets to treat pneumonia caused by Haemophilus parainfluenzae or Moraxella catarrhalis. Or, two 500-mg extended-release tablets PO daily × 7 d.† **Child:** 15 mg/kg

PO daily divided q 12 hr × 10 d (for *C. pneumoniae, Mycoplasma pneumoniae,* or *Streptococcus pneumoniae* only).†

➤ *Acute exacerbations of chronic bronchitis caused by* Moraxella catarrhalis, Streptococcus pneumoniae, Haemophilus influenzae, *or* Haemophilus parainfluenzae—**Adult:** 250 mg PO q 12 hr × 7-14 d (for *Moraxella catarrhalis* and *Streptococcus pneumoniae* only), or 500 mg PO q 12 hr × 7 d (up to 14 d for *Haemophilus influenzae*). Or, two 500-mg extended-release tablets PO daily × 7 d.†

➤ *Uncomplicated skin and skin-structure infections caused by* Staphylococcus aureus *or* Streptococcus pyogenes—**Adult:** 250 mg PO q 12 hr × 7-14 d.

➤ *Acute OM caused by* Haemophilus influenzae, Moraxella catarrhalis, *or* Streptococcus pneumoniae—**Child:** 7.5 mg/kg PO q 12 hr, up to 500 mg bid.†

---

clindamycin hydrochloride
Cleocin, Dalacin C*

clindamycin palmitate hydrochloride
Cleocin Pediatric, Dalacin C Palmitate*

clindamycin phosphate
Cleocin Phosphate, Cleocin T, Dalacin C Phosphate*

Lincomycin derivative; antibiotic
PRC: B

Available forms
Capsules: 75, 150, 300 mg; **hydrochloride, palmitate hydrochloride** *Granules for oral solution:* 75 mg/5 ml; **phosphate**

Injection: 150 mg base/ml, 300 mg base/2 ml, 600 mg base/4 ml, 900 mg base/6 ml; *Injection for IV infusion (in D₅W):* 300, 600, 900 (50 ml)

Indications & dosages
➤ *Infection*—**Adult:** 150-450 mg PO q 6 hr; or 300-600 mg IM or IV q 6, 8, or 12 hr. **Child > 1 mo:** 8-5 mg/kg PO daily in divided doses q 6-8 hr; or 15-40 mg/kg IM or IV daily in divided doses q 6 or 8 hr.

➤ *Endocarditis prophylaxis for dental procedures in patients allergic to PCN*—**Adult:** 600 mg PO 1 hr before procedure. **Child:** 20 mg/kg PO 1 hr before procedure.

➤ *PID*—**Adult:** 900 mg IV q 8 hr with gentamicin. Continue ≥ 48 hr after symptoms improve; then switch to 450 mg clindamycin PO qid for total course of 14 d.

---

clomipramine hydrochloride
Anafranil

TCA; antiobsessional drug
PRC: C

Available forms
Capsules: 25, 50, 75 mg

Indications & dosages
➤ *OCD*—**Adult:** 25 mg PO daily with meal; increase to 100 mg daily in divided doses over 1st 2 wk. Then, increase to max 250 mg daily in divided doses with meal prn. After adjustment, may give total doses hs. **Child:** 25 mg PO daily with meal; increase over 1st 2 wk to max

---

§ Adjust in immunocompromised patients

¶ Adjust in debilitated patients

3 mg/kg/d or 100 mg PO in divided doses, whichever is smaller. After adjustment, may give total doses hs. Max, 3 mg/kg/d or 200 mg/d, whichever is smaller.

clonazepam
Klonopin

Benzodiazepine; anticonvulsant
PRC: NR; CSS: IV

Available forms
Tablets: 0.5, 1, 2 mg

Indications & dosages
➤ *Lennox-Gastaut syndrome; atypical absence, akinetic, and myoclonic seizures*—**Adult:** 1.5 mg PO daily in 3 divided doses. Increase by 0.5-1 mg q 3 d until seizures are controlled. If given in unequal doses, give largest dose hs. Max, 20 mg/d. **Child ≤ 10 yr or 30 kg:** 0.01-0.03 mg/kg PO daily (max, 0.05 mg/kg/d), in 2-3 divided doses. Increase 0.25-0.5 mg q 3rd d to max maintenance dose, 0.1-0.2 mg/kg/d prn.

clonidine
Catapres-TTS

clonidine hydrochloride
Catapres, Dixarit*

Centrally acting adrenergic; antihypertensive
PRC: C

Available forms
clonidine *Transdermal:* TTS-1 (releases 0.1 mg/24 hr), TTS-2 (releases 0.2 mg/24 hr), TTS-3 (releases 0.3 mg/24 hr); **hydrochloride** *Tablets:* 0.025*, 0.1, 0.2, 0.3 mg

Indications & dosages
➤ *Essential and renal HTN*—**Adult:** 0.1 mg bid; may increase by 0.1 mg daily at wkly intervals. Usual dose range, 0.2-0.6 mg daily in 2-3 divided doses. Max, 2.4 mg daily.† Or, transdermal patch applied to nonhairy, intact skin on upper arm or torso q 7 d, starting with 0.1-mg system; then adjust with another 0.1-mg or larger system after 1-2 wk if desired response isn't achieved.†

clopidogrel bisulfate
Plavix

Adenosine diphosphate-induced platelet aggregation inhibitor; antiplatelet drug
PRC: B

Available forms
Tablets: 75 mg

Indications & dosages
➤ *Reduce atherosclerotic events in patients with recent CVA, MI, or peripheral arterial disease*—**Adult:** 75 mg PO daily.
➤ *Reduce atherosclerotic events in patients with acute coronary syndrome*—**Adult:** 300 mg PO × 1 dose; then 75 mg PO daily with 75-325 mg aspirin daily.

clorazepate dipotassium

Apo-Clorazepate*, Novo-Clopate*, Tranxene, Tranxene-SD, Tranxene T-Tab

Benzodiazepine; anxiolytic, anticonvulsant, sedative-hypnotic
PRC: D; CSS: IV

Available forms

Capsules: 3.75, 7.5, 15 mg; *Tablets:* 3.75, 7.5, 11.25, 15, 22.5 mg

Indications & dosages

➤ *Alcohol withdrawal*—**Adult:** On d 1, 30 mg PO in 1 dose; then 30-60 mg PO in divided doses; on d 2, 45-90 mg PO in divided doses; on d 3, 22.5-45 mg PO in divided doses; on d 4, 15-30 mg PO in divided doses; then reduce to 7.5-15 mg daily. Max, 90 mg daily.

➤ *Partial seizure disorder*—**Adult, child > 12 yr:** Max initial dose, 7.5 mg PO tid. Increase by ≤ 7.5 mg/wk to max 90 mg daily. **Child 9-12 yr:** Max initial dose, 7.5 mg PO bid. Increase by ≤ 7.5 mg/wk to max 60 mg daily.

clotrimazole

Canesten Vaginal*, Gyne-Lotrimin, Lotrimin, Mycelex, Mycelex-7, Mycelex-G, Mycelex OTC

Synthetic imidazole derivative; antifungal
PRC: B

Available forms

Combination pack: vaginal inserts 100, 200 mg and vulvar cream 1%; *Cream, topical lotion and solution, vaginal cream:* 1%; *Troche:* 10 mg; *Vaginal tablets:* 100, 200, 500 mg

Indications & dosages

➤ *Superficial fungal infection*—**Adult, child:** Apply thinly and massage into affected and surrounding area, am and pm, × 2-4 wk.

➤ *Vulvovaginal candidiasis*—**Adult:** Two 100-mg or one 200-mg vaginal tablet inserted daily hs × 3 d, or one 500-mg vaginal tablet daily hs × 1 d; or one applicator vaginal cream daily hs × 3-7 d.

➤ *Oropharyngeal candidiasis*—**Adult, child > 3 yr:** Dissolve troche over 15-30 min in mouth 5 times/d × 14 d.

➤ *Prevention of oropharyngeal candidiasis in immunocompromised patients*—**Adult, child:** Dissolve troche in mouth × 15-30 min tid during chemo or until corticosteroid therapy is reduced.

clozapine

Clozaril

Tricyclic dibenzodiazepine derivative; antipsychotic
PRC: B

Available forms

Tablets: 12.5, 25, 100 mg

Indications & dosages

➤ *Schizophrenia, reduce risk of recurrent suicidal behavior in schizophrenia or schizoaffective disorders*—**Adult:** 12.5 mg PO daily or bid; increase by 25-50 mg daily to 300-450 mg daily by end of 2 wk. Don't increase subsequent dose more than 1 or 2 times/wk; max, 100 mg/wk.

---

§ Adjust in immunocompromised patients   ¶ Adjust in debilitated patients

Usually, 300-600 mg daily; max, 900 mg/d. Assess regularly for agranulocytosis.

codeine phosphate
Paveral*

codeine sulfate

Opioid; analgesic, antitussive
PRC: C; CSS: II

Available forms
phosphate *Injection:* 30, 60 mg/ml; *Oral solution:* 15 mg/5 ml; *Tablets (solution):* 30, 60 mg; **sulfate** *Tablets (solution):* 15, 30, 60 mg

Indications & dosages
➤ *Pain*—**Adult:** 15-60 mg PO or 15-60 mg phosphate SC, IM, or IV q 4-6 hr prn. **Child > 1 yr:** 0.5 mg/kg PO, SC, or IM q 4 hr prn.
➤ *Cough*—**Adult:** 10-20 mg PO q 4-6 hr. Max, 120 mg/d. **Child 6-12 yr:** 5-10 mg PO q 4-6 hr; max, 60 mg/d. **Child 2-6 yr:** 2.5-5 mg PO q 4-6 hr; max, 30 mg/d.

colchicine

Alkaloid; antigout drug
PRC: C (PO), D (IV)

Available forms
Injection: 1 mg (⅟₆₀ grain)/2 ml; *Tablets:* 0.5 mg (⅟₁₂₀ grain), 0.6 mg (⅟₁₀₀ grain)

Indications & dosages
➤ *Gout prevention*—**Adult:** 0.5 or 0.6 mg PO. If attacks < 1/yr, give 3-4 d/week; if attacks > 1/yr, give daily.
➤ *Gout prevention in surgical patient*—**Adult:** 0.5 or 0.6 mg PO tid × 3 d preop and 3 d postop.
➤ *Acute gout, acute gouty arthritis*—**Adult:** 1-1.2 mg PO; then 0.5-0.6 mg q 1 hr or 1-1.2 mg q 2 hr until relief, nausea, vomiting, or diarrhea ensue or max dose of 8 mg is reached. Don't give additional doses of drug (PO) for at least 3 d. Or, 2 mg IV; then 0.5 mg IV q 6 hr prn. Max 4 mg/24 h. Don't give additional doses of drug (PO or IV) for at least 7 d.

colesevelam hydrochloride
Welchol

Polymeric bile acid sequestrant; antilipemic
PRC: B

Available forms
Tablets: 625 mg

Indications & dosages
➤ *Adjunct to diet and exercise, either alone or with an HMG-CoA reductase inhibitor, to reduce LDL level in patients with primary hypercholesterolemia (Frederickson type IIa)*—**Adult:** 3 tablets (1,875 mg) PO bid with meals and liq or 6 tablets (3,750 mg) once daily with meal and liq. May increase daily dosage to 7 tablets (4,375 mg) for added effect.

---

co-trimoxazole (trimethoprim and sulfamethoxazole)

Apo-Sulfatrim*, Bactrim DS, Septra, SMZ-TMP, Sulfatrim

Sulfonamide and folate antagonist; antibiotic
PRC: C (contraindicated at term)

Available forms

Injection: trimethoprim 16 mg and sulfamethoxazole 80 mg/ml in 5-, 10-, 20-, and 30-ml vials; *Oral suspension:* trimethoprim 40 mg and sulfamethoxazole 200 mg/5 ml; *Tablets (single strength):* trimethoprim 80 mg and sulfamethoxazole 400 mg; *Tablets (double strength):* trimethoprim 160 mg and sulfamethoxazole 800 mg

Indications & dosages

➤ *Shigellosis or UTI from Escherichia coli, Proteus, Klebsiella, or Enterobacter*—**Adult:** 1 DS tablet PO q 12 hr × 10-14 d for UTI and × 5 d for shigellosis. For uncomplicated cystitis or acute urethral syndrome, 1 DS tablet q 12 hr × 3 d. Or, IV infusion 8-10 mg/kg/d trimethoprim in 2-4 divided doses q 6, 8, or 12 hr ≤ 14 d for severe UTI. Max, 960 mg trimethoprim. **Child > 2 mo:** 8 mg/kg/d trimethoprim PO in 2 divided doses q 12 hr (10 d for UTI; 5 d for shigellosis). Or, IV infusion 8-10 mg/kg/d trimethoprim in 2-4 divided doses q 6, 8, or 12 hr. Don't exceed adult dose.†
➤ *Chronic bronchitis, upper respiratory infection*—**Adult:** 160 mg trimethoprim/800 mg sulfamethoxazole PO q 12 hr × 10-14 d.†
➤ *UTI with prostatitis*—**Adult:** 160 mg trimethoprim/800 mg sulfamethoxazole PO bid × 3-6 mo.†

cyanocobalamin (vitamin B₁₂)

Anacobin*, Bedoz*, Crystamine, Crysti-12, Cyanoject

hydroxocobalamin (vitamin B₁₂)

Hydro-Cobex, Hydro-Crysti-12, LA-12

H_2O-soluble vitamin; vitamin, nutritional supplement
PRC: NR

Available forms

cyanocobalamin *Injection:* 100, 1,000 mcg/ml; *Tablets:* 100, 500, 1,000, 5,000 mcg; **hydroxocobalamin** *Injection:* 1,000 mcg/ml

Indications & dosages

➤ *Vitamin B₁₂ deficiency*—**Adult:** 30 mcg hydroxocobalamin IM daily × 5-10 d. Maintenance, 100-200 mcg IM q mo. **Child:** 1-5 mg hydroxocobalamin over > 2 wk in doses of 100 mcg IM. Maintenance, 30-50 mcg/mo IM.
➤ *Pernicious anemia, vitamin B₁₂ malabsorption*—**Adult:** 1,000 mcg cyanocobalamin IM or SC daily × 6-7 d; then 1,000 mcg IM or SC q mo. **Child:** 10-50 mcg IM or SC daily × 5-10 d; then 100-250 mcg IM or SC q 2-4 wk.

---

§ Adjust in immunocompromised patients   ¶ Adjust in debilitated patients

➤ *Methylmalonic aciduria*—**Neonate:** 1,000 mcg cyanocobalamin IM daily.

cyclobenzaprine hydrochloride
Flexeril

TCA derivative; skeletal muscle relaxant
PRC: B

Available forms
Tablet: 5, 10 mg

Indications & dosages
➤ *Muscle spasm*—**Adult:** Initially, 5 mg PO tid; may increase to 10 mg PO tid. Max, 60 mg daily; max duration, 2-3 wk.‡
Elderly: May give 5 mg qid or bid.

dalteparin sodium
Fragmin

Low–molecular-weight heparin; anti-coagulant
PRC: B

Available forms
Syringe: 2,500, 5,000 anti-Factor Xa IU/0.2 ml; *Vial:* 10,000 anti-Factor Xa IU/ml

Indications & dosages
➤ *DVT prevention in abdominal surgery*—**Adult:** 2,500 IU SC daily, starting 1-2 hr preop; repeat daily × 5-10 d postop.
➤ *DVT prevention in hip surgery*—**Adult:** 2,500 IU SC ≤ 2 hr before surgery and 2nd dose 2,500 IU SC in pm of surgery,

≥ 6 hr after 1st dose. If surgery is in pm, omit 2nd dose on day of surgery. On 1st postop d, 5,000 IU SC daily × 5-10 d. Or, 5,000 IU SC in pm before surgery, then 5,000 IU SC daily starting in pm of day of surgery × 5-10 d postop.
➤ *Risk of thromboembolic complications due to severely restricted mobility during acute illness*—**Adult:** 5,000 IU SC once daily × 12-14 d.

daptomycin
Cubicin

Cyclic lipopeptide antibacterial; antibiotic
PRC: B

Available forms
Powder for injection: 250-, 500-mg vials

Indications & dosages
➤ *Complicated skin-structure infections*—**Adult:** 4 mg/kg IV infusion over 30 min q 24 hr × 7-14 d.†

darbepoetin alfa
Aranesp

Hematopoietic; antianemic
PRC: C

Available forms
Injection: 25, 40, 60, 100, 200, 300, 500 mcg/ml (albumin solution) in single-dose vials

Indications & dosages
➤ *Anemia related to chronic RF*—**Adult:** 0.45 mcg/kg IV or SC once/wk. Adjust

dose to avoid exceeding a target Hgb level of 12 g/dl. Don't increase dose more often than monthly. If Hgb level is increasing toward 12 g/dl, reduce dose by 25%. If level continues to increase, withhold dose until Hgb level begins to decrease, and then restart drug at a dose 25% below previous dose. If Hgb level increases by > 1 g/dl over 2 wk, decrease dose by 25%. If increase is < 1 g/dl over 4 wk and iron stores are adequate, increase dose by 25% of previous dose. Make further increases at 4-wk intervals until target Hgb is reached.

➤ *Anemia related to chemo*—**Adult:** 2.25 mcg/kg SC once/wk. If Hgb increases < 1 g/dl after 6 wk, increase dose up to 4.5 mcg/kg. If Hgb increases by more than 1 g/dl in a 2-wk period or if the Hgb exceeds 12 g/dl, reduce dose by approximately 25%. If Hgb exceeds 13 g/dl, withhold drug until Hgb drops to 12 g/dl, then restart at a dose approximately 25% below the previous dose.

delavirdine mesylate
Rescriptor

Nonnucleoside reverse-transcriptase inhibitor; antiretroviral
PRC: C

Available forms
Tablets: 100, 200 mg

Indications & dosages
➤ *HIV-1 infection*—**Adult:** 400 mg PO tid with other antiretrovirals.

desipramine hydrochloride
Norpramin

Dibenzazepine TCA; antidepressant
PRC: C

Available forms
Tablets (regular or film-coated): 10, 25, 50, 75, 100, 150 mg

Indications & dosages
➤ *Depression*—**Adult:** 100-200 mg PO daily in divided doses or hs; increase to max 300 mg daily. **Elderly, adolescent:** 25-100 mg PO daily in divided doses, up to max 150 mg daily.

desloratadine
Clarinex, Claritin Reditabs

Selective H_1-receptor antagonist; antihistamine
PRC: C

Available forms
Tablets: 5 mg; *Tablets (orally disintegrating):* 5 mg

Indications & dosages
➤ *Allergic rhinitis; chronic idiopathic urticaria*—**Adult, child ≥ 12 yr:** 5 mg PO daily.†, ‡

---

§ Adjust in immunocompromised patients   ¶ Adjust in debilitated patients

dexamethasone (injectable)
Decadron, Hexadrol

dexamethasone acetate
Cortastat LA, Dalalone D.P., Decaject-LA, Dexasone L.A., Dexone LA, Solurex LA

dexamethasone sodium phosphate
Dalalone, Decadron Phosphate, Dexasone

Glucocorticoid; anti-inflammatory, immunosuppressant
PRC: C

Available forms
dexamethasone *Elixir:* 0.5 mg/5 ml; *Oral solution:* 0.5 mg/5 ml, 1 mg/ml; *Tablets:* 0.25, 0.5, 0.75, 1, 1.5, 2, 4, 6 mg; **acetate** *Injection:* 8, 16 mg/ml suspension; **sodium phosphate** *Injection:* 4, 10, 20, 24 mg/ml

Indications & dosages
➤ *Cerebral edema*—**Adult:** 10 mg (phosphate) IV; then 4-6 mg IM q 6 hr; taper over 5-7 d.
➤ *Inflammation, allergic reactions, neoplasias*—**Adult:** 0.75-9 mg/d PO or 0.5-9 mg/d phosphate IM; or 4-16 mg acetate IM into joint or soft tissue q 1-3 wk; or 0.8-1.6 mg acetate into lesions q 1-3 wk.
➤ *Shock*—**Adult:** 1-6 mg/kg phosphate IV in 1 dose; or 40 mg IV q 2-6 hr prn.

dexamethasone (ophthalmic)
Maxidex

dexamethasone sodium phosphate
AK-Dex, Decadron

Corticosteroid; ophthalmic anti-inflammatory
PRC: C

Available forms
dexamethasone *Ophthalmic suspension:* 0.1%; **sodium phosphate** *Ophthalmic ointment:* 0.05%; *Ophthalmic solution:* 0.1%

Indications & dosages
➤ *Uveitis, iridocyclitis, inflammatory eye conditions, corneal injury, allergic conjunctivitis, suppression of graft rejection after keratoplasty*—**Adult, child:** 1 or 2 drops suspension or solution or 1.25-2.5 cm ointment into conjunctival sac. Initially, drops may be used from 6 times/d to q hr or ointment applied tid or qid depending on severity. Taper as condition improves.

dexmethylphenidate hydrochloride
Focalin

Methylphenidate derivative; CNS stimulant
PRC: C; CSS: II

Available forms
Tablets: 2.5, 5, 10 mg

Indications & dosages

➤ *ADHD*—**Child 6-17 yr:** For patients who aren't taking racemic methylphenidate, 2.5 mg PO bid, at least 4 hr apart. Adjust in wkly increments of 2.5-5 mg daily, to max 20 mg daily in divided doses. For patients taking methylphenidate, starting dose is ½ current methylphenidate dose. Max, 20 mg PO daily in divided doses.

diazepam
Apo-Diazepam*, Diazepam Intensol, Valium

Benzodiazepine; anxiolytic, skeletal muscle relaxant, amnestic, anticonvulsant, sedative-hypnotic
PRC: D; CSS: IV

Available forms
Injection: 5 mg/ml; *Oral solution:* 5 mg/5 ml; 5 mg/ml; *Tablets:* 2, 5, 10 mg

Indications & dosages

➤ *Anxiety*—**Adult:** 2-10 mg PO bid-qid. Or, 2-10 mg IM or IV q 3-4 hr prn. **Elderly:** 2-2.5 mg daily or bid; increase prn. **Child ≥ 6 mo:** 1-2.5 mg PO tid or qid; increase prn.

➤ *Muscle spasm*—**Adult:** 2-10 mg PO bid-qid. Or, 5-10 mg IM or IV, then 5-10 mg IM or IV q 3-4 hr prn. **Child ≥ 5 yr:** 5-10 mg IM or IV q 3-4 hr prn. **Child > 30 d-5 yr:** 1-2 mg IM or IV slowly; repeat q 3-4 hr prn.

➤ *Status epilepticus*—**Adult:** 5-10 mg IV (preferred) or IM. Repeat q 10-15 min prn, to a total dose of 30 mg. Repeat q 2-4 hr prn. **Child ≥ 5 yr:** 1 mg IV q 2-5 min

prn to total dose of 10 mg. Repeat q 2-4 hr prn. **Child > 30 d-5 yr:** 0.2-0.5 mg IV slowly q 2-5 min prn to total dose of 5 mg. Repeat q 2-4 hr prn.

diclofenac potassium
Cataflam

diclofenac sodium
Solaraze, Voltaren, Voltaren-ER, Voltaren SR*

NSAID; antiarthritic, anti-inflammatory
PRC: B

Available forms
Gel: 3%; *Suppository:* 50*, 100 mg*; *Tablets:* 50 mg; *Tablets (delayed-release):* 25, 50, 75 mg; *Tablets (extended-release):* 100 mg

Indications & dosages

➤ *Ankylosing spondylitis*—**Adult:** 25 mg delayed-release PO qid. An additional 25 mg dose may be needed hs.
➤ *OA*—**Adult:** 50 mg PO bid or tid, or 75 mg diclofenac potassium or delayed-release PO bid. Or 100 mg extended-release PO daily.
➤ *RA*—**Adult:** 50 mg PO tid or qid. Or, 75 mg diclofenac potassium or delayed-release PO bid. Or, 100 mg extended-release PO daily or bid.
➤ *Analgesia; primary dysmenorrhea*—**Adult:** 50 mg diclofenac potassium PO tid.
➤ *Actinic keratosis*—**Adult:** Apply gel to lesion bid.

dicyclomine hydrochloride
Antispas, Bentyl, Neoquess, Spasmoban*

Anticholinergic; antimuscarinic, GI antispasmodic
PRC: B

Available forms
Capsules: 10, 20 mg; *Injection:* 10 mg/ml; *Syrup:* 10 mg/5 ml; *Tablets:* 20 mg

Indications & dosages
➤ *IBS, functional GI disorders*—**Adult:** 20 mg PO qid; increase to 40 mg qid. Or 20 mg IM q 4-6 hr.

didanosine (ddl)
Videx, Videx EC

Purine analogue; antiviral
PRC: B

Available forms
Capsules (delayed-release): 125, 200, 250, 400 mg; *Powder for oral solution (buffered):* 100, 167, 250 mg/packet; *Powder for oral solution (pediatric):* 4-, 8-oz glass bottles contain 2, 4 g Videx, respectively; *Tablets (buffered, chewable):* 25, 50, 100, 150, 200 mg

Indications & dosages
➤ *HIV infection*—**Adult ≥ 60 kg:** 200 mg tablet PO q 12 hr; or 250 mg buffered powder PO q 12 hr; or 400 mg capsule PO daily. **Adult < 60 kg:** 125 mg tablet PO q 12 hr; or 167 mg buffered powder PO q 12 hr; or 250 mg capsule PO daily. **Child:** 120 mg/m² PO q 12 hr.†

digoxin
Digitek, Lanoxicaps, Lanoxin

Cardiac glycoside; antiarrhythmic, inotropic
PRC: C

Available forms
Capsules: 0.05, 0.1, 0.2 mg; *Elixir:* 0.05 mg/ml; *Injection:* 0.1 (pediatric), 0.25 mg/ml; *Tablets:* 0.125, 0.25 mg

Indications & dosages
➤ *HF, PSVT, atrial fibrillation and flutter*—**Adult:** Loading, 0.5-1 mg IV or PO in divided doses over 24 hr; maintenance, 0.125-0.5 mg IV or PO daily. **Adult > 65 yr:** Maintenance, 0.125 mg PO daily. **Premature neonate:** Loading, 0.015-0.025 mg/kg IV in 3 divided doses over 24 hr; maintenance, 0.01 mg/kg daily, divided q 12 hr. **Neonate:** Loading, 0.025-0.035 mg/kg PO, divided q 8 hr over 24 hr; or, IV loading 0.02-0.03 mg/kg; maintenance, 0.01 mg/kg PO daily, divided q 12 hr. **Child 1 mo-2 yr:** Loading, 0.035-0.06 mg/kg PO in 3 divided doses over 24 hr; or, IV loading, 0.03-0.05 mg/kg; maintenance, 0.01-0.02 mg/kg PO daily, divided q 12 hr. **Child > 2 yr:** Loading, 0.02-0.04 mg/kg PO daily, divided q 8 hr over 24 hr. Or, IV loading, 0.015-0.035 mg/kg; maintenance, 0.012 mg/kg PO daily, divided q 12 hr.†

---

digoxin immune Fab (ovine)
Digibind, DigiFab

Antibody fragment; cardiac glycoside antidote
PRC: C

Available forms
Injection: 38-, 40-mg vial

Indications & dosages
➤ *Digitalis intoxication*—**Adult, child:** Dose is highly specific; 1 vial binds about 0.5 mg of digoxin. Average dose, 10 vials.

diltiazem hydrochloride
Apo-Diltiaz*, Cardizem, Cardizem CD, Cardizem LA, Cardizem SR, Cartia XT, Dilacor XR, Diltia XT, Tiazac

Calcium channel blocker; antianginal
PRC: C

Available forms
Capsules (extended-release): 60, 90, 120, 180, 240, 300, 360, 420 mg; *Capsules (sustained-release):* 60, 90, 120 mg; *Injection:* 5 mg/ml (25 mg and 50 mg); *Tablets:* 30, 60, 90, 120 mg

Indications & dosages
➤ *Vasospastic angina, stable angina pectoris*—**Adult:** 30 mg PO qid ac and hs. Adjust prn over 1 or 2 d to max 360 mg/d in 3-4 divided doses. Or, 120 or 180 mg extended-release PO daily. Adjust prn over 7-14 d to max 480 mg daily.
➤ *HTN*—**Adult:** 60-120 mg PO bid tablets or sustained-release. Adjust prn to max 360 mg/d. Or, 180-240 mg daily extended-release. Adjust prn. Max, 540 mg/d. Or, 120-240 mg Cardizem LA PO daily at same time each day. Adjust q 14 d to max 540 mg/d.
➤ *Atrial fibrillation or flutter, PSVT*—**Adult:** 0.25 mg/kg as IV bolus injection over 2 min. If no response and no hypotension, 0.35 mg/kg IV after 15 min; then continue infusion 10 mg/hr (range, 5-15 mg/hr). Max infusion rate, 15 mg/hr.

diphenhydramine hydrochloride
Allerdryl*, Benadryl, Hydramine, Nytol Maximum Strength, Sominex

Ethanolamine-derivative antihistamine; antihistamine, antiemetic, antivertigo drug, antitussive, sedative-hypnotic, antidyskinetic
PRC: B

Available forms
Capsules: 25, 50 mg; *Elixir:* 12.5 mg/5 ml (14% alcohol); *Injection:* 50 mg/ml; *Syrup:* 12.5 mg/5 ml (5% alcohol); *Tablets, capsules:* 25, 50 mg; *Tablets (chewable):* 12.5 mg

Indications & dosages
➤ *Rhinitis, allergy symptoms, motion sickness, Parkinson's disease*—**Adult, child ≥ 12 yr:** 25-50 mg PO tid or qid; or 10-50 mg deep IM or IV. Max IM or IV dose, 400 mg/d. **Child < 12 yr:** 5 mg/kg daily PO, deep IM, or IV in divided doses qid. Max, 300 mg/d.
➤ *Sedation*—**Adult:** 25-50 mg PO or deep IM prn.

➤ *Cough*—**Adult:** 25 mg PO q 4-6 hr; max, 150 mg/d. **Child 6-12 yr:** 12.5 mg PO q 4-6 hr; max, 75 mg/d. **Child 2-6 yr:** 6.25 mg PO q 4-6 hr; max, 25 mg/d.

diphenoxylate hydrochloride and atropine sulfate
Logen, Lomanate, Lomotil, Lonox

Opioid; antidiarrheal
PRC: C; CSS: V

Available forms
Liq: 2.5 mg/5 ml (and atropine sulfate 0.025 mg/5 ml); *Tablets:* 2.5 mg (and atropine sulfate 0.025 mg)

Indications & dosages
➤ *Diarrhea*—**Adult:** 5 mg PO qid; adjust prn. **Child 2-12 yr:** 0.3-0.4 mg/kg liq form PO daily in 4 divided doses. Maintenance, reduce initial dose by up to 75% prn.

dipyridamole
IV Persantine, Persantine

Pyrimidine analogue; coronary vasodilator, platelet aggregation inhibitor
PRC: B

Available forms
Injection: 10 mg/2 ml; *Tablets:* 25, 50, 75 mg

Indications & dosages
➤ *To inhibit platelet adhesion in prosthetic heart valves*—**Adult:** 75-100 mg PO qid as adjunct to coumarin derivatives.

➤ *Alternative to exercise in CAD evaluation during thallium stress test*—**Adult:** 0.57 mg/kg IV infusion over 4 min (0.142 mg/kg/min).

dobutamine hydrochloride
Dobutrex

Adrenergic, beta$_1$-agonist; inotropic
PRC: B

Available forms
Injection: 12.5 mg/ml in 20-ml vials (parenteral)

Indications & dosages
➤ *To increase cardiac output caused by organic heart disease or from cardiac surgery*—**Adult:** 2.5-15 mcg/kg/min IV infusion. Increase prn to max 40 mcg/kg/min.

docetaxel
Taxotere

Taxoid; antineoplastic
PRC: D

Available forms
Injection: 20, 80 mg in single-dose vials

Indications & dosages
➤ *Breast CA*—**Adult:** 60-100 mg/m^2 IV over 1 hr q 3 wk. For patients who have febrile neutropenia, neutrophils < 500/mm^3 for > 1 wk, or severe or cumulative cutaneous reactions and who began therapy at 100 mg/m^2, decrease to 75 mg/m^2. If reactions continue, decrease dose to 55 mg/m^2 or stop therapy. For patients who began at 60 mg/m^2 without these re-

actions, dosage may be increased. Stop therapy in patients who develop ≥ grade 3 peripheral neuropathy.‡
► *Non–small-cell lung CA after platinum-based chemo has failed*—**Adult:** 75 mg/m² IV over 1 h q 3 wk. For patients who have febrile neutropenia, < 500/mm³ neutrophils for > 1 wk, severe or cumulative cutaneous reactions, or other grade 3/4 nonhematologic toxicities during treatment, withhold until toxicity resolves, then resume at 55 mg/m². Stop treatment in patients who develop ≥ grade 3 peripheral neuropathy.‡
► *With cisplatin, non–small-cell lung CA in patients who have not previously received chemo*—**Adult:** 75 mg/m² IV over 1 hr immediately followed by cisplatin 75 mg/m² over 30-60 min q 3 wk. In patients whose lowest platelet count during previous therapy was < 25,000/mm³, in those with febrile neutropenia, and in those with serious nonhematologic toxicity, decrease docetaxel dosage to 65 mg/m². In patients who need a further reduction, give 50 mg/m².‡

docosanol
Abreva

Aliphatic alcohol; antiviral
PRC: B

Available forms
Cream: 10%

Indications & dosages
► *Recurrent oral-facial herpes simplex*—**Adult, child ≥ 12 yr:** Apply topically 5 times/d starting with first symptoms; con-tinue until lesion is healed; rub in gently but completely.

docusate calcium
Surfak

docusate sodium
Colace, Diocto liquid, Diocto syrup, D-S-S

Surfactant; emollient laxative
PRC: C

Available forms
calcium *Capsules:* 240 mg; **sodium** *Capsules:* 50, 100, 250 mg; *Oral liq:* 150 mg/15 ml; *Syrup:* 20 mg/5 ml, 50, 60 mg/15 ml, 100 mg/30 ml; *Tablets:* 100 mg

Indications & dosages
► *Stool softening*—**Adult, child > 12 yr:** 50-500 mg PO daily until BM is normal. **Child < 3 yr:** 10-40 mg sodium PO daily. **Child 3-6 yr:** 20-60 mg sodium PO daily. **Child 6-12 yr:** 40-120 mg sodium PO daily.

dofetilide
Tikosyn

Antiarrhythmic; class III antiarrhythmic
PRC: C

Available forms
Capsules: 125, 250, 500 mcg

Indications & dosages
► *To maintain normal sinus rhythm (NSR) in patients who had symptomatic atrial fibrillation or flutter for > 1 wk; con-

---

§ Adjust in immunocompromised patients   ¶ Adjust in debilitated patients

version of atrial fibrillation or flutter to NSR—**Adult:** 500 mcg PO bid if CrCl is > 60 ml/min; 250 mcg PO bid if CrCl is 40-60 ml/min; 125 mcg PO bid if CrCl is 20-40 ml/min. Measure QTc interval before 1st dose and q 2 or 3 hr after each dose in hospital. If QTc interval increases > 15% or is > 500 milliseconds (550 milliseconds in ventricular conduction abnormalities) 2-3 hr after 1st dose, adjust as follows: If initial dose was 500 mcg PO bid, give 250 mcg PO bid. If initial dose was 250 mcg PO bid, give 125 mcg PO bid. If initial dose was 125 mcg PO bid, give 125 mcg PO daily. If QTc interval is > 500 milliseconds (550 milliseconds in ventricular conduction abnormalities) any time after 2nd dose, stop drug.

dolasetron mesylate
Anzemet

Selective serotonin 5-HT$_3$–receptor antagonist; antinauseant, antiemetic
PRC: B

Available forms
Injection: 20 mg/ml as 12.5 mg/0.625-ml ampule or 100 mg/5-ml vial; *Tablets:* 50, 100 mg

Indications & dosages
➤ *To prevent nausea and vomiting in chemo*—**Adult:** 100 mg PO 1 hr before chemo; or 1.8 mg/kg (or fixed dose of 100 mg) IV 30 min before chemo. **Child 2-16 yr:** 1.8 mg/kg PO 1 hr before chemo; or 1.8 mg/kg IV 30 min before chemo.
➤ *To prevent postop nausea and vomiting*—**Adult:** 100 mg PO ≤ 2 hr preop;

12.5 mg IV 15 min before anesthesia ends. **Child 2-16 yr:** 1.2 mg/kg PO ≤ 2 hr preop; max,100 mg. Can mix injection with apple or apple-grape juice and give PO; max, 100 mg. Or, 0.35 mg/kg (max, 12.5 mg) IV 15 min before anesthesia ends.
➤ *Postop nausea and vomiting*—**Adult:** 12.5 mg IV when symptoms occur. **Child 2-16 yr:** 0.35 mg/kg (max,12.5 mg) IV when symptoms occur.

donepezil hydrochloride
Aricept

Acetylcholinesterase inhibitor; Alzheimer's disease drug
PRC: C

Available forms
Tablets: 5, 10 mg

Indications & dosages
➤ *Dementia (Alzheimer's type)*—**Adult:** 5 mg PO daily hs. After 4-6 wk, may increase to 10 mg daily.

dopamine hydrochloride
Intropin, Revimine*

Adrenergic; inotropic, vasopressor
PRC: C

Available forms
Injection: 40, 80, 160 mg/ml parenteral concentrate for injection for IV infusion; 0.8 mg/ml (200 or 400 mg), 1.6 mg/ml (400 or 800 mg), 3.2 mg/ml (800 mg) in D$_5$W parenteral injection for IV infusion

---

Indications & dosages
➤ *Shock, to improve perfusion to vital organs, to increase cardiac output, hypotension*—**Adult:** 1-5 mcg/kg/min IV infusion. Increase infusion by 1-4 mcg/kg/min q 10-30 min prn.

dorzolamide hydrochloride
Trusopt

Sulfonamide; antiglaucoma drug
PRC: C

Available forms
Ophthalmic solution: 2%

Indications & dosages
➤ *To increase IOP in patients with ocular HTN or open-angle glaucoma*—**Adult:** 1 drop in affected eye tid.

doxazosin mesylate
Cardura

Alpha blocker; antihypertensive
PRC: C

Available forms
Tablets: 1, 2, 4, 8 mg

Indications & dosages
➤ *HTN*—**Adult:** 1 mg PO daily; evaluate standing and supine BP at 2-6 hr and 24 hr after dose. Increase slowly to 2 mg, 4 mg, then 8 mg daily prn. Max, 16 mg.
➤ *BPH*—**Adult:** 1 mg PO daily in am or pm; may increase to 2 mg, then 4 mg, and 8 mg daily prn. Adjust q 1-2 wk.

doxepin hydrochloride
Adapin, Novo-Doxepin*, Sinequan, Triadapin*

TCA; antidepressant
PRC: NR

Available forms
Capsules: 10, 25, 50, 75, 100, 150 mg; *Oral concentrate:* 10 mg/ml

Indications & dosages
➤ *Depression, anxiety*—**Adult:** Initially, 25-75 mg PO daily or in divided doses. Increase to max 300 mg daily. Maintenance, usually 75-150 mg/d. If giving entire maintenance dose once daily, max is 150 mg.

doxycycline calcium
Vibramycin

doxycycline hyclate
Apo-Doxy*, Doryx, Doxy-100, Doxy-200, Doxycin*, Doxytec*, Novo-Doxylin*, Nu-Doxycycline*, Periostat, Vibramycin, Vibra-Tabs

doxycycline monohydrate
Adoxa, Monodox, Vibramycin

Tetracycline; antibiotic
PRC: D

Available forms
calcium *Oral suspension:* 50 mg/5 ml; **hyclate** *Capsules:* 20, 50, 100 mg; *Capsules (enteric-coated pellets):* 75, 100 mg; *Injection:* 100, 200 mg; *Tablets:* 20, 100 mg; **monohydrate** *Capsules:* 50, 100 mg; *Oral*

suspension: 25 mg/5 ml; *Tablets:* 50, 75, 100 mg

Indications & dosages

➤ *Acute gonococcal infection*—200 mg PO × 1 dose followed with 100 mg at hs on d 1, then 100 mg PO bid × 3 d. Or, 300 mg PO × 1 dose; repeat 300 mg PO in 1 hr.

➤ *Infection from susceptible gram-pos and gram-neg organisms,* Rickettsia, Mycobacterium pneumoniae, Chlamydia trachomatis, *and* Borrelia burgdorferi; *psittacosis; granuloma inguinale*—**Adult, child > 8 yr or ≥ 45 kg:** 100 mg PO q 12 hr on d 1; then 100 mg PO daily; or 200 mg IV on d 1 in 1-2 infusions; then 100-200 mg IV daily. **Child > 8 yr or < 45 kg:** 4.4 mg/kg PO or IV daily in divided doses q 12 hr on d 1; then 2.2-4.4 mg/kg daily in 1-2 divided doses. Give IV infusion ≥ 1 hr.

➤ *Urethral, endocervical, or rectal infection from* C. trachomatis *or* U. urealyticum—**Adult:** 100 mg PO bid ≥ 7 d (10 d for epididymitis).

➤ *PID*—**Adult:** 100 mg IV q 12 hr; continue ≥ 2 d after symptoms improve; then 100 mg PO q 12 h × total 14 d.

➤ *Adjunct to other antibiotics for inhalation, GI, and oropharyngeal anthrax*—**Adult:** 100 mg q 12 hr IV initially until susceptibility tests are known. Switch to 100 mg PO bid when appropriate. Treat × 60 d total. **Child > 8 yr and > 45 kg:** 100 mg q 12 hr IV, then switch to 100 mg PO bid when appropriate. Treat × 60 d total. **Child > 8 yr and ≤ 45 kg:** 2.2 mg/kg q 12 hr IV, then switch to 2.2 mg/kg PO bid when appropriate. Treat × 60 d total.

Child ≤ 8 yr: 2.2 mg/kg 12 hr IV, then switch to 2.2 mg/kg PO bid when appropriate. Treat × 60 d total.

➤ *Cutaneous anthrax*—**Adult:** 100 mg PO bid × 60 d. **Child > 8 yr and > 45 kg:** 100 mg PO q 12 hr × 60 d. **Child > 8 yr and ≤ 45 kg:** 2.2 mg/kg PO q 12 hr × 60 d. **Child ≤ 8 yr:** 2.2 mg/kg q 12 hr PO × 60 d.

➤ *Periodontitis*—**Adult:** 20 mg Periostat PO bid > 1 hr before or 2 hr after am and pm meals and after scaling and root planing. Effective for 9 mo.

droperidol
Inapsine

Dopamine blocker, butyrophenone derivative; antipsychotic, neuroleptic
PRC: C

Available forms
Injection: 2.5 mg/ml in 1-, 2-ml ampule and 2-ml vials

Indications & dosages
➤ *To reduce the risk of nausea and vomiting during surgical and diagnostic procedures*—**Adult, child > 12 yr:** 2.5-10 mg IM or IV. May give additional 1.25 mg, prn. **Child 2-12 yr:** Max initial dose, 0.1 mg/kg. Adjust dose in elderly and patients taking depressants.¶

➤ *Delirium*—**Adult:** 5 mg IV.

---

drotrecogin alfa (activated)
Xigris

Recombinant human activated protein C; anti-infective
PRC: C

Available forms
Injection: 5-, 20-mg vials

Indications & dosages
➤ **Severe sepsis**—**Adult:** 24 mcg/kg/hr IV infusion × 96 hr.

dutasteride
Avodart

5-Alpha-reductase enzyme inhibitor; BPH drug
PRC: X

Available forms
Capsules: 0.5 mg

Indications & dosages
➤ **BPH**—**Man:** 0.5 mg PO daily.

efalizumab
Raptiva

Immunosuppressant; anti-psoriatic
PRC: C

Available forms
Injection: 125-mg single-use vial

Indications & dosages
➤ **Plaque psoriasis**—**Adult:** Single dose of 0.7 mg/kg SC; follow 1 wk later with wkly doses of 1 mg/kg SC. Max, 200 mg.

efavirenz
Sustiva

Nonnucleoside reverse transcriptase inhibitor; antiretroviral
PRC: C

Available forms
Capsules: 50, 100, 200 mg; *Tablets:* 600 mg

Indications & dosages
➤ *HIV-1 infection, given with protease inhibitor or nucleoside analogue reverse transcriptase inhibitor*—**Adult:** 600 mg PO daily. **Child ≥ 3 yr or ≥ 40 kg:** 600 mg PO daily. **Child ≥ 3 yr or 10 kg to < 40 kg:** If 10 to < 15 kg, give 200 mg PO daily; 15 to < 20 kg, 250 mg PO daily; 20 to < 25 kg, 300 mg PO daily; 25 to < 32.5 kg, 350 mg PO daily; 32.5 to < 40 kg, 400 mg PO daily.

eflornithine hydrochloride
Vaniqa

Ornithine decarboxylase inhibitor; hair growth retardant
PRC: C

Available forms
Cream: 13.9%

Indications & dosages
➤ *Reduction of unwanted facial hair*—**Woman, girl ≥ 12 yr:** Apply thin layer to affected facial areas and adjacent areas under chin and rub in thoroughly bid, at least 8 hr apart.

---

§ Adjust in immunocompromised patients   ¶ Adjust in debilitated patients

eletriptan hydrobromide
Relpax

Serotonin 5-HT₁ receptor agonist; anti-migraine drug
PRC: C

Available forms
Tablets: 20, 40 mg

Indications & dosages
➤ *Migraines—***Adult:** 20-40 mg PO taken at first sign of migraine attack. If headache recurs after initial relief, may repeat dose in ≥ 2 hr. Max, 80 mg/d, max single dose, 40 mg.

emtricitabine
Emtriva

Nucleoside reverse transcriptase inhibitor; antiretroviral
PRC: B

Available forms
Capsules: 200 mg

Indications and dosages
➤ *HIV-1 infection, given with other antiretrovirals—***Adult:** 200 mg PO daily.†

enalaprilat

enalapril maleate

ACE inhibitor; antihypertensive
PRC: C (D, 2nd and 3rd trimesters)

Available forms
enalaprilat *Injection:* 1.25 mg/ml;
enalapril maleate *Tablets:* 2.5, 5, 10, 20 mg

Indications & dosages
➤ *HTN—***Adult:** For patients not on diuretics, 2.5-5 mg PO daily, then adjust prn. Range 10-40 mg daily in 1 dose or 2 divided doses. Or, 1.25 mg IV q 6 hr over 5 min. For patients on diuretics, 2.5 mg PO daily. Or, 0.625 mg IV over 5 min; repeat in 1 hr prn, then 1.25 mg IV q 6 hr.†
➤ *To switch from IV to PO—***Adult:** 5 mg PO daily; for patients who had been receiving 0.625 mg IV q 6 hr, then 2.5 mg PO daily.†
➤ *To switch from PO to IV—***Adult:** 1.25 mg IV over 5 min q 6 hr.†

enfuvirtide
Fuzeon

HIV-1 and CD4 fusion inhibitor; anti-HIV drug, antiviral
PRC: B

Available forms
Injection: 108-mg single-use vials (90 mg/ml after reconstitution)

Indications & dosages
➤ *HIV-1 infection, with other antiretrovirals—***Adult:** 90 mg SC bid; inject into the upper arm, anterior thigh, or abdomen. **Child 6-16 yr:** 2 mg/kg SC bid; max, 90 mg/dose.

enoxaparin sodium
Lovenox

Low-molecular-weight heparin; anti-coagulant
PRC: B

Available forms
Injection: 30 mg/0.3 ml, 40 mg/0.4 ml, 60 mg/0.6 ml, 80 mg/0.8 ml, 100 mg/ml, 120 mg/0.8 ml, 150 mg/ml

Indications & dosages
➤ *To prevent DVT, which may lead to PE, following hip or knee replacement surgery*—**Adult:** 30 mg SC q 12 hr × 7-10 d. Initial dose between 12 and 24 hr postop if hemostasis is established.
➤ *To prevent DVT, which may lead to PE, after abdominal surgery*—**Adult:** 40 mg SC daily × 7-10 d. Initial dose 2 hr before surgery.
➤ *To prevent ischemic complications of unstable angina and non-Q-wave MI, when given with aspirin*—**Adult:** 1 mg/kg SC q 12 hr × 2-8 d, with aspirin PO.
➤ *To lessen risk of embolism from decreased mobility during acute illness*—**Adult:** 40 mg daily SC × 6-11 d. Up to 14 d has been well tolerated.
➤ *DVT in inpatients with or without PE, with warfarin*—**Adult:** 1 mg/kg SC q 12 hr; or 1.5 mg/kg SC daily × 5-7 d until INR is 2-3. Start warfarin sodium ≥ 72 hr after enoxaparin.
➤ *DVT in outpatients without PE, with warfarin sodium*—**Adult:** 1 mg/kg SC q 12 hr × 5-7 d until INR is 2-3. Start warfarin sodium ≤ 72 hr after enoxaparin.

entacapone
Comtan

Catechol-O-methyltransferase inhibitor; antiparkinsonian
PRC: C

Available forms
Tablets: 200 mg

Indications & dosages
➤ *Parkinson's disease*—**Adult:** 200 mg PO with each dose of levodopa-carbidopa. Max, 8 doses/d (1,600 mg/d).

epinastine hydrochloride
Elestat

Histamine receptor antagonist, mast cell stabilizer; ophthalmic antihistamine
PRC: C

Available forms
Ophthalmic solution: 0.05% in 5-and 10-ml bottles

Indications & dosages
➤ *To prevent itching associated with allergic conjunctivitis*—**Adult, child ≥ 3:** Instill 1 drop into each eye bid. Continue as long as allergen is present, even if patient has no symptoms.

---

§ Adjust in immunocompromised patients   ¶ Adjust in debilitated patients

epinephrine (adrenaline)
Adrenalin, Bronkaid Mist, Primatene Mist Mistometer*, Primatene Mist

epinephrine bitartrate
AsthmaHaler Mist, Bronkaid Suspension Mist

epinephrine hydrochloride
Adrenalin Chloride, AsthmaNefrin*, EpiPen, EpiPen Jr., Racepinephrine, Sus-Phrine, Vaponefrin

Adrenergic; bronchodilator, vasopressor, cardiac stimulant
PRC: C

Available forms
Aerosol inhalation: 160, 200, 220, 250 mcg/metered spray; *Injection:* 0.01 (1:100,000), 0.1 (1:10,000), 0.5 (1:2,000), 1 (1:1,000) mg/ml, 5 mg/ml (1:200) parenteral suspension; *Nebulizer inhalation:* 1% (1:100)*, 1.25%*, 2.25%*

Indications & dosages
➤ *Bronchospasm, hypersensitivity reactions, anaphylaxis*—**Adult:** 0.1-0.5 ml 1:1,000 SC or IM. Repeat q 10-15 min prn. Or, 0.1-0.25 ml 1:1,000 IV over 5-10 min. **Child:** 0.01 ml (10 mcg) 1:1,000/kg SC; repeat q 20 min-4 hr prn. Or, 0.004-0.005 ml/kg 1:200 Sus-Phrine SC; repeat q 8-12 hr prn.
➤ *Acute asthma attack*—**Adult, child ≥ 4 yr:** 160-250 mcg (metered aerosol), equivalent to 1 inhalation, repeated × 1 dose prn, after 1 min; no subsequent doses for ≥ 3 hr. Or, 1% (1:100) solution

epinephrine or 2.25% solution racepinephrine by hand-bulb nebulizer as 1-3 deep inhalations; repeat q 3 hr prn.
➤ *Cardiac arrest*—**Adult:** 0.5-1 mg IV. Repeat q 3-5 min prn. Higher-dose epinephrine: 3-5 mg (about 0.1 mg/kg) repeated q 3-5 min. **Child:** 0.01 mg/kg (0.1 ml/kg 1:10,000 injection) IV. ET tube: 0.1 mg/kg (0.1 ml/kg 1:1,000 injection) diluted in 1-2 ml ½ NSS or NSS. Subsequent IV or intratracheal doses 0.1-0.2 mg/kg (0.1-0.2 ml/kg 1:1,000 injection). May repeat q 3-5 min.

eplerenone
Inspra

Aldosterone receptor antagonist; antihypertensive
PRC: B

Available forms
Tablets: 25, 50, 100 mg

Indications & dosages
➤ *HTN*—**Adult:** 50 mg PO daily. Increase to 50 mg PO bid after 4 wk, if response is inadequate. Max, 100 mg daily. In patients taking weak CYP 3A4 inhibitors (erythromycin, fluconazole, saquinavir, verapamil), reduce eplerenone starting dose to 25 mg PO once daily.
➤ *HF post-MI*—**Adult:** 25 mg PO daily. Adjust within 4 wk as tolerated to 50 mg PO once daily. Increase to 50 mg PO daily within 4 wk as tolerated. If potassium level < 5 mEq/L, increase from 25 mg q other d to 25 mg/d, or increase from 25 mg/d to 50 mg/d. If potassium level is

5-5.4 mEq/L, don't adjust dosage. If potassium level is 5.5-5.9 mEq/L, decrease from 50 mg/d to 25 mg/d, or decrease from 25 mg/d to 25 mg q other d, or if dosage was 25 mg q other d, withhold drug. If potassium level > 6 mEq/L, withhold drug. May restart drug at 25 mg q other d when potassium level < 5.5 mEq/L.

epoetin alfa (erythropoietin)
Epogen, Procrit

Glycoprotein; antianemic
PRC: C

Available forms
Injection: 2,000, 3,000, 4,000, 10,000 units/ml; multidose vials of 10,000, 20,000 units/ml

Indications & dosages
➤ *Anemia in end-stage renal disease*—**Adult:** 50-100 units/kg IV 3 times/wk (SC or IV in non-hemodialysis patients). Reduce dose when target Hct is reached or Hct rises > 4 points in 2-wk period. Increase dose if Hct doesn't increase by 5-6 points after 8 wk of therapy.
➤ *HIV-infected patients with anemia, secondary to zidovudine therapy*—**Adult:** 100 units/kg IV or SC 3 times/wk × 8 wk or target Hgb level is reached. After 8 wk, may increase by 50-100 units/kg IV or SC 3 times/wk prn. After 4-8 wk, may increase in increments of 50-100 units/kg 3 times/wk; max, 300 units/kg IV or SC 3 times/wk.

➤ *Anemia, secondary to chemo*—**Adult:** 150 units/kg SC 3 times/wk × 8 wk or target Hgb level is reached.

eprosartan mesylate
Teveten

Angiotensin II receptor antagonist; antihypertensive
PRC: C (D, 2nd and 3rd trimesters)

Available forms
Tablets: 400, 600 mg

Indications & dosages
➤ *HTN*—**Adult:** 600 mg PO daily. Range, 400-800 mg daily in 1 dose or divided bid.

ertapenem
Invanz

Carbapenem; anti-infective
PRC: B

Available forms
Injection: 1 g

Indications & dosages
➤ *Complicated intra-abdominal infections caused by* Escherichia coli, Clostridium clostridiiforme, Eubacterium lentum, Peptostreptococcus *species,* Bacteroides fragilis, B. distasonis, B. ovatus, B. thetaiotaomicron, B. uniformis—**Adult:** 1 g IV or IM daily × 5-14 d.†
➤ *Complicated skin and skin-structure infections caused by* Staphylococcus aureus *(methicillin-susceptible strains),* Streptococcus pyogenes, Escherichia coli,

---

§ Adjust in immunocompromised patients ¶ Adjust in debilitated patients

Peptostreptococcus *species*—**Adult:** 1 g IV or IM daily × 7-14 d.†

➤ *Community-acquired pneumonia caused by* Streptococcus pneumoniae *(penicillin-susceptible strains),* Haemophilus influenzae *(beta-lactamase–negative strains),* Moraxella catarrhalis—**Adult:** 1 g IV or IM daily × 10-14 d. If improvement after ≥ 3 d, switch to PO to complete full course.†

➤ *Complicated UTIs, including pyelonephritis caused by* Escherichia coli, Klebsiella pneumoniae—**Adult:** 1 g IV or IM daily × 10-14 d. If improvement after ≥ 3 d, switch to PO to complete full course.†

➤ *Acute pelvic infections including postpartum endomyometritis, septic abortion, and postsurgical gynecologic infections caused by* Streptococcus agalactiae, Escherichia coli, B. fragilis, Porphyromonas asaccharolyticus, Peptostreptococcus *species,* Prevotella bivia—**Adult:** 1 g IV or IM daily × 3-10 d.†

erythromycin base
Apo-Erythro base*, E-Base, E-Mycin, Erybid*, Eryc, Ery-Tab, Erythromycin Base Filmtab, Erythromycin Delayed-Release, PCE Dispertab

erythromycin estolate
Ilosone, Ilosone Pulvules

erythromycin ethylsuccinate
Apo-Erythro-ES*, E.E.S., E.E.S. Granules, EryPed, EryPed 200, EryPed 400

erythromycin lactobionate
Erythrocin

erythromycin stearate
Apo-Erythro-S, Erythrocin Stearate

Erythromycin; antibiotic
PRC: B

Available forms
base *Capsules (delayed-release, enteric-coated):* 250 mg; *Tablets (enteric-coated):* 250, 333, 500 mg; *Tablets (filmtabs):* 250, 500 mg; **estolate** *Capsules:* 250 mg; *Oral suspension:* 125, 250 mg/5 ml; *Tablets:* 500 mg; **ethylsuccinate** *Oral suspension:* 200, 400 mg/ml; 100 mg/2.5 ml; *Tablets (film-coated):* 400 mg; *Powder for oral suspension:* 200 mg/5 ml, 400 mg/5 ml; **lactobionate** *Injection:* 500-mg, 1-g vial; **stearate** *Tablets (film-coated):* 250, 500 mg

Indications & dosages
➤ *PID from* Neisseria gonorrhoeae—**Adult:** 500 mg IV lactobionate q 6 hr × 3 d, then 250 mg base, estolate, or stearate; or 400 mg ethylsuccinate PO q 6 hr × 7 d.

➤ *Respiratory tract, skin, soft-tissue infection*—**Adult:** 250-500 mg base, estolate, or stearate PO q 6 hr; or 400-800 mg ethylsuccinate PO q 6 hr; or 15-20 mg/kg IV daily lactobionate continuous infusion or divided doses q 6 hr × 10 d. **Child:** 30-50 mg/kg PO daily, divided doses q 6 hr; or 15-20 mg/kg IV daily divided doses q 4-6 hr × 10 d.

---

escitalopram oxalate
Lexapro

SSRI; antidepressant
PRC: C

Available forms
Solution: 5 mg/5 ml; *Tablets:* 5, 10, 20 mg

Indications & dosages
➤ *Major depressive disorder*—**Adult:**
10 mg PO daily; increase to 20 mg prn,
after ≥ 1 wk. **Elderly:** 10 mg PO daily.‡
➤ *8-week therapy for generalized anxiety
disorder*—**Adult:** Initially, 10 mg PO once
daily. May increase to 20 mg daily after a
minimum of 1 wk.

esmolol hydrochloride
Brevibloc

Beta blocker; antiarrhythmic
PRC: C

Available forms
Injection: 10-mg/ml vial; 250-mg/ml ampule

Indications & dosages
➤ *SVT, atrial fibrillation or flutter, non-
compensatory ST; postop HTN*—**Adult:**
Loading dose, 500 mcg/kg/min IV infusion over 1 min; then 4-min maintenance
infusion of 50 mcg/kg/min. If no response
in 5 min, repeat loading dose, then maintenance infusion of 100 mcg/kg/min ×
4 min. Repeat loading dose and increase
maintenance infusion by 50-mcg/kg/min
increments. Max maintenance infusion for

tachycardia, 25-200 mcg/kg/min. May
need up to 300 mcg/kg/min for HTN.
➤ *Intraop tachycardia or HTN*—**Adult:**
80 mg (about 1 mg/kg) IV bolus over
30 sec; then 150 mcg/kg/min IV infusion
prn. Adjust rate prn. Max, 300 mcg/kg/
min.

esomeprazole magnesium
Nexium

*Proton pump inhibitor, s-isomer of
omeprazole; gastroesophageal drug*
PRC: B

Available forms
*Capsules (delayed-release containing
enteric-coated pellets):* 20, 40 mg (sup-
plied as 22.3 or 44.5 mg esomeprazole
magnesium)

Indications & dosages
➤ *GERD, healing of erosive esophagitis*—
Adult: 20 or 40 mg PO daily × 4-8 wk.‡
➤ *Maintenance of healing in erosive
esophagitis*—**Adult:** 20 mg PO daily ×
≥ 6 mo.‡
➤ *Symptomatic GERD*—**Adult:** 20 mg PO
daily × 4 wk. If symptoms continue,
treatment may continue × 4 more wk.‡
➤ *Eradication of* Helicobacter pylori, *with
other drugs, to reduce duodenal ulcer
recurrence*—**Adult:** 40 mg PO daily with
amoxicillin 1,000 mg PO bid and clarithromycin 500 mg PO bid, all × 10 d.‡

esterified estrogens
Estratab, Menest, Neo-Estrone*

Estrogen; estrogen replacement, antineoplastic
PRC: X

Available forms
Tablets, tablets (film-coated): 0.3, 0.625, 1.25, 2.5 mg

Indications & dosages
➤ *Inoperable prostate CA*—**Men:** 1.25-2.5 mg PO tid.
➤ *Breast CA*—**Men and postmenopausal women:** 10 mg PO tid ≥ 3 mo.
➤ *Hypogonadism*—**Women:** 2.5-7.5 mg daily in divided doses in cycles of 20 d on, 10 d off.
➤ *Castration, primary ovarian failure*—**Women:** 1.25 mg daily in cycles of 3 wk on, 1 wk off. Adjust prn.
➤ *Osteoporosis prevention*—**Postmenopausal women:** 0.3-1.25 mg daily.

estradiol
Alora, Climara, Esclim, Estraderm, Vivelle, Vivelle Dot

estradiol cypionate
Depo-Estradiol

estradiol hemihydrate
Estrasorb

estradiol valerate
Climara, Delestrogen, Dioval, Estradiol L.A., Estra-L 40, Gynogen L.A., Menaval-20

Estrogen; estrogen replacement, antineoplastic
PRC: X

Available forms
estradiol *Tablets (micronized):* 0.5, 1, 2 mg; *Transdermal:* 0.025, 0.0375 mg, 0.05 mg, 0.06 mg, 0.075 mg, 0.1 mg/24 hr, 4 mg/10 cm^2 (delivers 0.05 mg/24 hr), 8 mg/20 cm^2 (delivers 0.1 mg/24 hr); *Vaginal cream (in non-liquefying base):* 0.1 mg/g; **cypionate** *Injection (in oil):* 5 mg/ml; **hemihydrate** *Topical emulsion:* 4.35 mg estradiol hemihydrate/1.74 g; 3.48 g of emulsion delivers 0.05 mg estradiol/day; **valerate** *Injection (in oil):* 10, 20, 40 mg/ml

Indications & dosages
➤ *Menopausal symptoms, hypogonadism, castration, primary ovarian failure*—**Women:** 1-2 mg PO estradiol daily in cycles of 21 d on, 7 d off, or cycles of 5 d on, 2 d off. Or, 0.025-mg/d system (Esclim) or 0.05-mg/d system (Estraderm) applied twice/wk. Or, 0.05-mg/d system (Climara) once/wk. Or, 1-5 mg cypionate IM q 3-4 wk, or 10-20 mg valerate IM q 4 wk prn.
➤ *Menopausal symptoms*—**Women:** Apply contents of two 1.74-g foil pouches (total 3.48 g) hemihydrate to left thigh and calf daily. Rub until thoroughly absorbed; rub excess emulsion remaining on hands onto the buttocks. Let dry before covering with clothing.

➤ *Breast CA*—**Men and postmenopausal women:** 10 mg PO estradiol tid × 3 mo.

➤ *Prostate CA*—**Men:** 30 mg IM valerate q 1-2 wk; or 1-2 mg PO estradiol tid.

➤ *Osteoporosis prevention*—**Postmenopausal women:** 0.025-mg/d system (Alora, Vivelle, Vivelle Dot). Or, 0.05-mg/d system (Estraderm) applied to clean, dry area of trunk twice/wk. Or, 0.025-mg/d system (Climara) once/wk.

estrogens, conjugated (estrogenic substances, conjugated)
C.E.S.*, Premarin, Premarin Intravenous, Cenestin

Estrogen; estrogen replacement, antineoplastic, antiosteoporotic
PRC: X

Available forms
Injection: 25 mg/5 ml; *Tablets:* 0.3, 0.45, 0.625, 0.9, 1.25, 2.5 mg; *Vaginal cream:* 0.625 mg/g

Indications & dosages
➤ *Abnormal uterine bleeding*—**Women:** 25 mg IV or IM; repeat in 6-12 hr prn.

➤ *Castration, primary ovarian failure*—**Women:** 1.25 mg PO daily in cycles of 3 wk on, 1 wk off. Adjust dose prn.

➤ *Osteoporosis*—**Postmenopausal women:** 0.3-0.625 mg PO daily in cycles of 3 wk on, 1 wk off.

➤ *Vulvar or vaginal atrophy*—**Women:** 0.5-2 g cream intravaginally once daily in cycles of 3 wk on, 1 wk off. Or, 0.3 mg PO daily.

➤ *Hypogonadism*—**Women:** 0.3 to 0.625 mg daily in cycles of 3 wk on, 1 wk off.

➤ *Palliative treatment of inoperable prostate CA*—**Men:** 1.25-2.5 mg PO tid.

➤ *Palliative treatment of breast CA*—**Adult:** 10 mg PO tid × ≥ 3 mo.

estropipate (piperazine estrone sulfate)
Ogen, Ortho-Est

Estrogen; estrogen replacement
PRC: X

Available forms
Tablets: 0.75, 1.5, 3, 6 mg; *Vaginal cream:* 1.5 mg/g

Indications & dosages
➤ *Primary ovarian failure, castration, hypogonadism*—**Women:** 1.25-7.5 mg PO daily × 1st 3 wk, then rest × 8-10 d. If no bleeding occurs by end of rest, repeat cycle.

➤ *Vasomotor menopausal symptoms*—**Women:** 0.625-5 mg PO daily in cycles of 3 wk on, 1 wk off.

➤ *To prevent osteoporosis*—**Women:** 0.625 mg PO daily × 25 d of 31-d cycle.

etanercept
Enbrel

Fusion protein; antirheumatic
PRC: B

Available forms
Injection: 25-mg single-use vial

---

§ Adjust in immunocompromised patients ¶ Adjust in debilitated patients

Indications & dosages
➤ *RA, psoriatic arthritis, ankylosing spondylitis*—**Adult:** 50 mg SC wkly, given as two 25-mg injections at separate sites either on the same day or 72-96 hr apart.
➤ *Juvenile RA*—**Child 4-17 yr:** 0.8 mg/kg SC wkly (max, 50 mg/wk) given either on 1 d or divided in 2 injections given 72-96 hr apart. Max of 25 mg/dose may be given at a single injection site.

ethambutol hydrochloride
Etibi*, Myambutol

Semisynthetic antituberculotic; antituberculotic
PRC: B

Available forms
Tablets: 100, 400 mg

Indications & dosages
➤ *Pulmonary TB*—**Adult, child > 13 yr:** 15 mg/kg PO daily. Retreatment, 25 mg/kg PO daily × 60 d (or smears, cultures negative) with at least 1 other antituberculotic; then decrease to 15 mg/kg/d.

etodolac
Lodine

NSAID; antiarthritic
PRC: C

Available forms
Capsules: 200, 300 mg; *Tablets:* 400, 500 mg; *Tablets (extended-release):* 400, 500, 600 mg

Indications & dosages
➤ *Pain*—**Adult:** 200-400 mg PO q 6-8 hr prn; max, 1,200 mg daily. For patients ≤ 60 kg, max is 20 mg/kg/d.

ezetimibe
Zetia

Selective cholesterol absorption inhibitor; antihypercholesterolemic
PRC: C

Available forms
Tablets: 10 mg

Indications & dosages
➤ *Adjunct to diet and exercise to reduce cholesterol, LDL, and apolipoprotein-B levels in patients with primary hypercholesterolemia, alone or combined with HMG-CoA reductase inhibitors or bile acid sequestrants; adjunct to other lipid-lowering drugs in patients with homozygous familial hypercholesterolemia; adjunct to diet in patients with homozygous sitosterolemia to reduce sitosterol and campesterol levels*—**Adult:** 10 mg PO daily.

famciclovir
Famvir

Synthetic acyclic guanine derivative; antiviral
PRC: B

Available forms
Tablets: 125, 250, 500 mg

Indications & dosages

➤ *Herpes zoster (shingles)*—**Adult:** 500 mg PO q 8 hr × 7 d.†

➤ *Recurrent genital herpes*—**Adult:** 125 mg PO bid × 5 d. Start when symptoms occur.†

famotidine
Pepcid, Pepcid AC, Pepcid RPD

H_2-receptor antagonist; antiulcerative
PRC: B

Available forms

Gelcaps: 10 mg; *Injection:* 10 mg/ml; *Powder for oral suspension:* 40 mg/ml after reconstitution; *Premixed injection:* 20 mg/50 ml NSS; *Tablets:* 10, 20, 40 mg; *Tablets (chewable):* 10 mg; *Tablets (orally disintegrating):* 20, 40 mg

Indications & dosages

➤ *Duodenal ulcer*—**Adult:** 40 mg PO q hs, or 20 mg PO bid. Maintenance, 20 mg PO q hs.

➤ *Benign gastric ulcer*—**Adult:** 40 mg PO q hs × 8 wk.

➤ *GERD*—**Adult:** 20 mg PO bid ≤ 6 wk.

➤ *Esophagitis from GERD*—**Adult:** 20-40 mg bid × ≤ 12 wk.

➤ *Heartburn*—**Adult:** 10 mg Pepcid AC PO 1 hr ac for prevention or 10 mg Pepcid AC PO with H_2O for symptoms. Max, 20 mg daily. Don't give daily > 2 wk.

➤ *Hospitalized patient who has ulcerations or hypersecretory conditions, or who can't take drugs PO*—**Adult:** 20 mg IV q 12 hr.

felodipine
Plendil, Renedil*

Calcium channel blocker; antihypertensive
PRC: C

Available forms

Tablets (extended-release): 2.5, 5, 10 mg

Indications & dosages

➤ *HTN*—**Adult:** 5 mg PO daily. Adjust q 2 wk prn. Max, 20 mg daily. **Elderly > 65 yr:** 2.5 mg PO daily. Max, 10 mg daily.‡

fenofibrate
Lofibra, Tricor

Fibric acid derivative; antihyperlipidemic
PRC: C

Available forms

Micronized capsules: 67, 134, 200 mg; *Tablets:* 54, 160 mg

Indications & dosages

➤ *Hypertriglyceridemia*—**Adult:** 54-160 mg tablets PO daily. Or, 67-200 mg capsules PO daily. Based on response, increase dose at 4- to 8-wk intervals to max 160 mg (tablets) or 200 mg (capsules) daily.† **Elderly:** Start treatment at 54 mg tablets PO daily or 67 mg capsules PO daily.†

➤ *Primary hypercholesterolemia or mixed hyperlipidemia*—**Adult:** 160 mg (tablets) PO daily. Or, 200 mg capsules PO daily.† **Elderly:** Start treatment at 54 mg tablets PO daily or 67 mg capsules PO daily and increase only after effects on

---

§ Adjust in immunocompromised patients   ¶ Adjust in debilitated patients

renal function and triglyceride level have been evaluated at this dose.†

fentanyl citrate
Sublimaze

fentanyl transdermal system
Duragesic

fentanyl transmucosal
Actiq

Opioid agonist; analgesic, adjunct to anesthesia, anesthetic
PRC: C; CSS: II

Available forms
Injection: 50 mcg/ml; *Lozenges:* 200, 400, 600, 800, 1,200, 1,600 mcg; *Transdermal system:* 25, 50, 75, 100 mcg/hr

Indications & dosages
➤ *Preop anesthesia*—**Adult:** 50-100 mcg IM 30-60 min preop.
➤ *Adjunct to general anesthesia*—**Adult:** Low-dose, 2 mcg/kg IV; moderate, 2-20 mcg/kg IV, then 25-100 mcg IV prn; high, 20-50 mcg/kg IV, then 25 mcg to ½ initial loading dose IV prn.
➤ *Adjunct to regional anesthesia*—**Adult:** 50-100 mcg IM or IV over 1-2 min prn.
➤ *Induction and maintenance of anesthesia*—**Child 2-12 yr:** 2-3 mcg/kg IV.
➤ *Postop pain*—**Adult:** 50-100 mcg IM q 1-2 hr prn.
➤ *Chronic pain*—**Adult:** 1 transdermal system applied to unirritated and unirradiated upper torso skin. Initially, 25-mcg/hr system × 72 hr (q 48 hr prn); adjust dose prn.
➤ *Breakthrough CA pain in opioid-tolerant patients:* Initially, 200 mcg Actiq lozenge; if no relief, repeat 15 min after first lozenge dissolves. Max, 2 lozenges per breakthrough pain episode. May increase prn until single lozenge provides adequate analgesia per breakthrough pain episode, but limit use to ≤ 4 daily.

ferrous gluconate
Fergon, Simron

Oral iron supplement; hematinic
PRC: A

Available forms
100 mg ferrous gluconate = 11.6 mg elemental iron
Tablets: 240, 325 mg

Indications & dosages
➤ *Iron deficiency*—**Adult:** 100-200 mg (2-3 mg/kg) elemental iron PO in 3 divided doses. **Child 2-12 yr:** 50-100 mg (1-1.5 mg/kg) elemental iron PO in 3-4 divided doses. **Child 6 mo-2 yr:** Up to 6 mg/kg/d PO in 3-4 divided doses. **Infant:** 10-25 mg in 3-4 divided doses PO.

ferrous sulfate
Apo-Ferrous Sulfate*, Feosol, Mol-Iron

ferrous sulfate, dried
Feosol

Oral iron supplement; hematinic
PRC: A

Available forms

Ferrous sulfate = 20% elemental iron; dried and powdered, about 32% elemental iron
Capsules: 250 mg; *Capsules (extended-release):* 160 mg (dried); *Drops:* 75 mg/0.6 ml, 125 mg/ml; *Elixir:* 220/5 ml; *Syrup:* 90 mg/5 ml; *Tablets:* 324, 325, 200 (dried) mg; *Tablets (extended-release):* 160 mg (dried)

Indications & dosages

➤ *Iron deficiency*—**Adult:** 100-200 mg (2-3 mg/kg) elemental iron PO in 3 divided doses. **Child 2-12 yr:** 50-100 mg (1-1.5 mg/kg) elemental iron PO in 3-4 divided doses. **Child 6 mo-2 yr:** Up to 6 mg/kg/d PO in 3-4 divided doses. **Infant:** 10-25 mg PO in 3-4 divided doses.

fexofenadine
Allegra

H_1-*receptor antagonist; antihistamine*
PRC: C

Available forms

Tablets: 30, 60, 180 mg

Indications & dosages

➤ *Seasonal allergic rhinitis*—**Adult, child ≥ 12 yr:** 60 mg PO bid or 180 mg PO once daily.† **Child 6-11 yr:** 30 mg PO bid.†
➤ *Chronic idiopathic urticaria*—**Adult, child ≥ 12 yr:** 60 mg PO bid.† **Child 6-11 yr:** 30 mg PO bid.†

filgrastim (granulocyte colony-stimulating factor; G-CSF)
Neupogen

Biologic response modifier; colony-stimulating factor
PRC: C

Available forms

Injection: 300 mcg/ml

Indications & dosages

➤ *To decrease incidence of infection in patients with non-myeloid malignant disease on myelosuppressive antineoplastics*—**Adult, child:** 5 mcg/kg/d IV or SC ≥ 24 hr after cytotoxic chemo. Increase by 5 mcg/kg for each chemo cycle based on neutrophil count.
➤ *To decrease incidence of infection in patients with non-myeloid malignant disease on myelosuppressive antineoplastics followed by bone marrow transplantation*—**Adult, child:** 10 mcg/kg/d IV or SC ≥ 24 hr after cytotoxic chemo and bone marrow infusion. Adjust dose based on neutrophil response.
➤ *Congenital neutropenia*—**Adult:** 6 mcg/kg SC bid. Adjust dose prn.

finasteride
Propecia, Proscar

Steroid (synthetic 4-azasteroid) derivative; androgen synthesis inhibitor
PRC: X

Available forms

Tablets: 1, 5 mg

§ Adjust in immunocompromised patients   ¶ Adjust in debilitated patients

Indications & dosages
➤ *Symptomatic BPH*—**Adult:** 5 mg Proscar PO daily.
➤ *Male-pattern hair loss*—**Man:** 1 mg Propecia PO daily.

flecainide acetate
Tambocor

Benzamide derivative local anesthetic; ventricular antiarrhythmic
PRC: C

Available forms
Tablets: 50, 100, 150 mg

Indications & dosages
➤ *PSVT; paroxysmal atrial fibrillation, flutter; supraventricular arrhythmias*—**Adult:** 50 mg PO q 12 hr. Increase 50 mg bid q 4 d prn. Max, 300 mg daily.
➤ *Life-threatening ventricular arrhythmias*—**Adult:** 100 mg PO q 12 hr. Increase 50 mg bid q 4 d prn. Max, 400 mg daily.†

fluconazole
Diflucan

Bis-triazole derivative; antifungal
PRC: C

Available forms
Injection: 200 mg/100 ml; 400 mg/200 ml; Powder for oral suspension: 10, 40 mg/ml; Tablet: 50, 100, 150, 200 mg

Indications & dosages
➤ *Oropharyngeal, esophageal candidiasis*—**Adult:** 200 mg PO or IV d 1; then 100 mg daily. Continue ≥ 2 wk after symptoms end. **Child:** 6 mg/kg on d 1; then 3 mg/kg ≥ 2 wk.†
➤ *Vaginal candidiasis*—**Adult:** 150 mg PO × 1 dose.†
➤ *Systemic candidiasis*—**Adult:** Up to 400 mg PO or IV daily. Continue ≥ 2 wk after symptoms end.†
➤ *Cryptococcal meningitis*—**Adult:** 400 mg PO or IV on d 1; then 200 mg daily. Continue 10-12 wk after CSF cultures are negative.†

fludrocortisone acetate
Florinef

Mineralocorticoid, glucocorticoid; mineralocorticoid replacement therapy
PRC: C

Available forms
Tablets: 0.1 mg

Indications & dosages
➤ *Adrenal insufficiency, salt-losing adrenogenital syndrome*—**Adult:** 0.1-0.2 mg PO daily. Decrease to 0.05 mg daily if transient HTN occurs. **Child:** 0.05-0.1 mg PO daily.
➤ *Orthostatic hypotension in diabetic patients, orthostatic hypotension*—**Adult:** 0.1-0.4 mg PO daily.

flumazenil
Romazicon

Benzodiazepine antagonist; antidote
PRC: C

Available forms

Injection: 0.1 mg/ml in 5-, 10-ml multi-dose vials

Indications & dosages

➤ *To reverse sedative effects of benzodiazepines*—**Adult:** 0.2 mg IV over 15 sec. After 45 sec, repeat at 1-min intervals until total dose of 1 mg is given (initial dose and 4 doses) prn; usually 0.6-1 mg. If resedation, may repeat after 20 min. Max, 1 mg at one time and 3 mg/hr.

➤ *Suspected benzodiazepine overdose*—**Adult:** 0.2 mg IV over 30 sec. After 30 sec, 0.3 mg given over 30 sec prn. If poor response, 0.5 mg over 30 sec; repeat 0.5-mg doses prn, at 1-min intervals until total dose of 3 mg. Usually 1-3 mg; rarely, patients may need more doses. Max, 5 mg. If resedation, may repeat after 20 min. Max 1 mg at one time and 3 mg/hr.

fluorouracil (5-fluorouracil, 5-FU)
Adrucil, Carac, Efudex, Fluoroplex

Antimetabolite (cell cycle–phase specific, S phase); antineoplastic
PRC: D (injection), X (topical)

Available forms

Cream: 1, 5%; *Injection:* 50 mg/ml; *Topical solution:* 1, 2, 5%

Indications & dosages

➤ *Colon, rectal, breast, stomach, pancreatic CA*—**Adult:** 12 mg/kg IV daily × 4 d; if no toxicity, 6 mg/kg on d 6, 8, 10, and 12; then single wkly maintenance dose of 10-15 mg/kg IV after toxicity subsides. Max single dose, 800 mg/d.

➤ *Advanced colorectal CA*—**Adult:** 425 mg/m² IV daily × 5 d. Give with 20 mg/m² leucovorin IV. Repeat at 4-wk intervals for 2 additional courses; repeat at intervals of 4-5 wk if tolerated.

➤ *Superficial basal cell CA*—**Adult:** Apply cream (5%) or topical solution (5%) bid × 3-6 wk.

➤ *Multiple actinic or solar keratosis of face and anterior scalp*—**Adult:** Wash and dry lesion area; wait 10 min. Apply thin layer to lesions daily for up to 4 wk.

fluoxetine hydrochloride
Prozac, Prozac Weekly, Sarafem

SSRI; antidepressant
PRC: C

Available forms

Capsules: 10, 20, 40 mg; *Capsules (delayed-release):* 90 mg; *Oral solution:* 20 mg/5 ml; *Tablets:* 10, 20 mg

Indications & dosages

➤ *Depression*—**Adult:** 20 mg Prozac PO q am; increase doses prn. Give doses > 20 mg bid. Max, 80 mg daily.† ‡ **Elderly:** 20 mg PO q am.† ‡ **Child 8-18 yr:** 10 mg PO daily. After 1 wk, increase to 20 mg daily. For lower-weight children, wait several wk before increasing dose.† ‡

➤ *Maintenance treatment for depression in stabilized patients*—**Adult:** 90 mg PO Prozac Weekly once/wk. Initiate once/wk-dosing 7 d after last daily dose of Prozac 20 mg.† ‡

---

§ Adjust in immunocompromised patients ¶ Adjust in debilitated patients

➤ *OCD*—**Adult:** 20 mg Prozac PO q am; increase dose prn. Give doses > 20 mg bid. Max, 80 mg daily.†, ‡ **Child 7-17 yr:** 10 mg PO daily. After 2 wk, increase dose to 20 mg/d. Dosage range, 20-60 mg/d. For lower-weight children increase to 20-30 mg/d after several wk. Max, 60 mg daily.†, ‡

➤ *Bulimia nervosa*—**Adult:** 60 mg PO Prozac q am.†, ‡

➤ *Short-term treatment of panic disorder*—**Adult:** 10 mg Prozac PO daily × 1 wk, then increase dose prn to 20 mg daily. Max, 60 mg daily.

➤ *PMDD*—**Adult:** 20 mg Sarafem PO daily continuously or intermittently (starting 14 d before anticipated onset of menstruation through the first full day of menses). Max, 80 mg daily.†, ‡

fluphenazine decanoate
Modecate*, Prolixin Decanoate

fluphenazine enanthate

fluphenazine hydrochloride
Moditen HCl*

Phenothiazine; antipsychotic
PRC: NR

Available forms
decanoate, enanthate *Depot injection:* 25 mg/ml; **hydrochloride** *IM injection:* 2.5 mg/ml; *Tablets:* 1, 2.5, 5, 10 mg

Indications & dosages
➤ *Psychotic disorders*—**Adult:** 0.5-10 mg PO daily in divided doses q 6-8 hr; increase to 20 mg prn. Maintenance, 1-

5 mg PO daily. For IM, give ⅓ to ½ of PO doses (usual, 1.25 mg). Initial range, 2.5-10 mg IM daily in divided doses q 6-8 hr. Use doses > 10 mg/d cautiously. Or, 12.5-25 mg of long-acting esters (decanoate) IM or SC q 1-6 wk; maintenance, 25-100 mg prn. **Elderly:** 1-2.5 mg hydrochloride daily.

fluticasone propionate (inhalation)
Flovent Inhalation Aerosol, Flovent Rotadisk

Corticosteroid; anti-inflammatory
PRC: C

Available forms
Oral inhalation aerosol: 44, 110, 220 mcg; *Oral inhalation powder:* 50, 100, 250 mcg

Indications & dosages
➤ *Asthma*—**Adult, child ≥ 12 yr:** If previously using bronchodilators only, Inhalation Aerosol dose of 88 mcg bid; max, 440 mcg bid. For patient previously using inhalation corticosteroids, Inhalation Aerosol dose of 88-220 mcg bid; max, 440 mcg bid. For patient previously using PO corticosteroids, Inhalation Aerosol dose of 880 mcg bid. Or, for patient previously using bronchodilators only, Rotadisk inhalation dose of 100 mcg bid; max, 500 mcg bid. For patient previously using inhalation corticosteroids, Rotadisk inhalation dose of 100-250 mcg bid; max 500 mcg bid. For patient previously using PO corticosteroids: Rotadisk inhalation dose of 1,000 mcg bid. **Child 4-11 yr:** For patient previously using bronchodilators

only or inhalation corticosteroids, Rotadisk inhalation dose of 50 mcg bid; max, 100 mcg bid.

fluticasone propionate (nasal)
Flonase

Corticosteroid; topical anti-inflammatory
PRC: C

Available forms
Nasal spray: 50 mcg/metered spray (16-g bottles)

Indications & dosages
➤ *Nasal symptoms of seasonal and perennial allergic and nonallergic rhinitis*—**Adult:** 2 sprays in each nostril daily or 1 spray bid. Maintenance, 1 spray in each nostril daily. Or, for seasonal allergic rhinitis, 2 sprays in each nostril daily prn. **Child ≥ 4 yr:** 1 spray in each nostril daily. May increase to 2 sprays in each nostril daily; then decrease to 1 spray in each nostril daily based on response. Max 2 sprays in each nostril daily.

fluvastatin sodium
Lescol, Lescol XL

HMG-CoA reductase inhibitor; antilipemic
PRC: X

Available forms
Capsules: 20, 40 mg; *Tablets (extended-release):* 80 mg

Indications & dosages
➤ *Primary hypercholesterolemia, mixed dyslipidemia, to slow progression of coronary atherosclerosis, to reduce risks from undergoing coronary revascularization procedures*—**Adult:** For patients requiring LDL reduction to a goal of ≥ 25%, initially, 40 mg regular-release and 80 mg extended-release as a single dose in the pm. Or, 40 mg regular-release PO bid. For patients requiring LDL reduction to a goal of < 25%, initially, 20 mg PO daily. Recommended range, 20-80 mg daily.‡

fluvoxamine maleate
Luvox

SSRI; antidepressant
PRC: C

Available forms
Tablets: 25, 50, 100 mg

Indications & dosages
➤ *OCD*—**Adult:** 50 mg PO daily hs; increase in 50-mg increments q 4-7 d prn. Max 300 mg daily. If total daily dose > 100 mg, give in 2 divided doses. **Elderly:** Use a lower initial dose and slower dose adjustment.† **Child 8-17 yr:** 25 mg PO hs. Increase in 25-mg increments q 4 to 7 d until max benefit. Max, 200 mg for children 8-11 yr; 300 mg for children 11-17 yr. Give total daily doses > 50 mg in 2 divided doses.†

folic acid
Folvite, Novo-Folacid*

Folic acid derivative; vitamin supplement
PRC: A

Available forms

Injection: 10-ml vials (5 mg/ml with 1.5% benzyl alcohol, 5 mg/ml with 1.5% benzyl alcohol and 0.2% EDTA); *Tablets:* 0.4, 0.8, 1 mg

Indications & dosages

➤ *RDA*—**Man, boy ≥ 11 yr:** 150-200 mcg. **Woman, girl ≥ 11 yr:** 150-180 mcg. **Child 7-10 yr:** 100 mcg. **Child 4-6 yr:** 75 mcg. **Birth-3 yr:** 25-50 mcg. **Pregnant woman:** 400 mcg. **Breastfeeding woman:** 260-280 mcg.
➤ *Megaloblastic or macrocytic anemia*—**Adult, child ≥ 4 yr:** 0.4-1 mg PO, SC, or IM daily. After correcting anemia, give proper diet and RDA supplements. **Child < 4 yr:** Up to 0.3 mg PO, SC, or IM daily. **Pregnant or breast-feeding woman:** 0.8 mg PO, SC, or IM daily.
➤ *To prevent megaloblastic anemia*—**Pregnant woman:** Up to 1 mg PO, SC, or IM daily.

fondaparinux sodium
Arixtra

Activated factor X (Xa) inhibitor; anticoagulant
PRC: B

Available forms

Injection: 2.5 mg/0.5 ml single-dose prefilled syringe

Indications & dosages

➤ *To prevent DVT in patients having hip fracture, hip replacement, or knee replacement surgery*—**Adult:** 2.5 mg SC daily × 5-9 d; max, 11 d. Give initial dose after hemostasis is established, 6-8 hr after surgery.

formoterol fumarate inhalation powder
Foradil Aerolizer

Long-acting selective beta$_2$ blocker; bronchodilator
PRC: C

Available forms

Capsules for inhalation: 12 mcg

Indications & dosages

➤ *Prevention and maintenance for bronchospasm in patients with reversible obstructive airway disease or nocturnal asthma who usually need treatment with short-acting inhaled beta$_2$-adrenergic agonists*—**Adult, child ≥ 5 yr:** One 12-mcg capsule by inhalation via Aerolizer inhaler q 12 hr. If symptoms are present between doses, use short-acting beta$_2$-adrenergic agonist for immediate relief.
➤ *To prevent exercise-induced bronchospasm*—**Adult, child ≥ 12 yr:** One 12-mcg capsule by inhalation via Aerolizer inhaler at least 15 min before exercise, given occasionally prn. Avoid giving additional doses within 12 hr of 1st dose.
➤ *Maintenance therapy for COPD*—**Adult:** One 12-mcg capsule q 12 hr using the Aerolizer inhaler.

fosamprenavir calcium
Lexiva

HIV protease inhibitor; antiretroviral
PRC: C

Available forms
Tablets: 700 mg

Indications & dosages
➤ *HIV infection*—**Adult:** In patients not previously treated, 1,400 mg PO bid without ritonavir. Or, 1,400 mg PO once daily and ritonavir 200 mg PO once daily. Or, 700 mg PO bid and ritonavir 100 mg PO bid. In patients previously treated with a protease inhibitor, 700 mg PO bid plus ritonavir 100 mg PO bid.‡ If the patient receives efavirenz, fosamprenavir, and ritonavir once daily, give an additional 100 mg/d of ritonavir (300 mg total).

foscarnet sodium (phosphonoformic acid)
Foscavir

Pyrophosphate analogue; antiviral
PRC: C

Available forms
Injection: 24 mg/ml in 250-, 500-ml bottles

Indications & dosages
➤ *CMV retinitis in AIDS patients*—**Adult:** For induction treatment, 60 mg/kg IV infusion over at least 1 hr q 8 hr × 2-3 wk or 90 mg/kg infusion over 1.5-2 hr q 12 hr × 2-3 wk. Then maintenance infusion of 90-120 mg/kg/d over 2 hr.†

➤ *Mucocutaneous acyclovir-resistant HSV*—**Adult:** 40 mg/kg IV over at least 1 hr q 8-12 hr × 2-3 wk.†

fosinopril sodium
Monopril

ACE inhibitor; antihypertensive
PRC: C (D, 2nd and 3rd trimesters)

Available forms
Tablets: 10, 20, 40 mg

Indications & dosages
➤ *HTN*—**Adult:** 10 mg PO daily. Adjust based on BP peak and trough levels. Usual dose, 20-40 mg. Max, 80 mg daily; may be divided. **Child 6-16 yr, > 50 kg:** 5-10 mg PO once daily.
➤ *HF*—**Adult:** 10 mg PO daily. Increase over several wk to max 40 mg PO daily.

fosphenytoin sodium
Cerebyx

Hydantoin derivative; anticonvulsant
PRC: D

Available forms
Injection: 2 ml (150 mg fosphenytoin sodium = 100 mg phenytoin sodium), 10 ml (750 mg fosphenytoin sodium = 500 mg phenytoin sodium)

Indications & dosages
➤ *Status epilepticus*—**Adult:** 15-20 mg phenytoin sodium equivalent (PE)/kg IV at 100-150 mg PE/min as loading dose; then 4-6 mg PE/kg/d IV as maintenance. (Phenytoin may be used instead.)

§ Adjust in immunocompromised patients   ¶ Adjust in debilitated patients

➤ *Seizures during neurosurgery*—**Adult:** Loading dose, 10-20 mg PE/kg IM or IV at rate ≤ 150 mg PE/min. Maintenance, 4-6 mg PE/kg/d IV.

➤ *Short-term substitution for PO phenytoin*—**Adult:** Same total daily dose equivalent as PO phenytoin in 1 dose daily IM or IV at ≤ 150 mg PE/min. May require more frequent dosing.

frovatriptan succinate
Frova

5-HT₁ receptor agonist; antimigraine drug
PRC: C

Available forms
Tablets: 2.5 mg

Indications & dosages
➤ *Migraine*—**Adult:** 2.5 mg PO. May repeat dose in ≥ 2 hr if migraine returns. Max, 7.5 mg daily.

fulvestrant
Faslodex

Estrogen receptor antagonist; antineoplastic
PRC: D

Available forms
Injection: 50 mg/ml in 2.5-ml and 5-ml prefilled syringes

Indications & dosages
➤ *Hormone-receptor–positive metastatic breast CA in postmenopausal women with disease progression following anti-estrogen therapy*—**Adult:** 250 mg by slow IM injection into buttock q mo.

furosemide
Apo-Furosemide*, Lasix, Novosemide*

Loop diuretic; diuretic, antihypertensive
PRC: C

Available forms
Injection: 10 mg/ml; *Oral solution:* 10 mg/ml, 40 mg/5 ml; *Tablets:* 20, 40, 80 mg

Indications & dosages
➤ *Pulmonary edema*—**Adult:** 40 mg IV over 1-2 min; then 80 mg IV in 1-1½ hr prn.
➤ *Edema*—**Adult:** 20-80 mg PO daily in am, 2nd dose in 6-8 hr; adjust to 600 mg daily prn. Or, 20-40 mg IM or IV; increase by 20 mg q 2 hr prn. Give IV dose slowly over 1-2 min. **Infant, child:** 2 mg/kg PO daily; increase by 1-2 mg/kg in 6-8 hr prn; adjust to 6 mg/kg/d prn.
➤ *HTN*—**Adult:** 40 mg PO bid. Adjust dose prn.

gabapentin
Neurontin

1-Aminomethyl cyclohexaneacetic acid; anticonvulsant
PRC: C

Available forms
Capsules: 100, 300, 400 mg; *Solution:* 250 mg/5 ml; *Tablets:* 600, 800 mg

---

Indications & dosages

➤ *Partial seizures*—**Adult:** 300 mg PO hs on d 1; 300 mg PO bid on d 2; then 300 mg PO tid on d 3. Increase prn to 1,800 mg/d in 3 divided doses. Max, 3,600 mg/d.†

➤ *Adjunct to control partial seizures*—**Child 3-12 yr:** 10-15 mg/kg/d PO in 3 divided doses initially; adjust over 3 d to reach these effective dosages: for child 5-12 yr, 25 to 35 mg/kg/d PO in 2 divided doses. For a child 3-4 yr: 40 mg/kg/d PO in 2 divided doses.†

➤ *Postherpetic neuralgia*—**Adult:** 300 mg PO on d 1, then 300 mg bid on d 2; 300 mg tid on d 3. Max, 1,800 mg daily in 3 divided doses.†

---

galantamine hydrobromide
Reminyl

Reversible competitive acetylcholinesterase inhibitor; cholinomimetic
PRC: B

Available forms

Oral solution: 4 mg/ml; *Tablets:* 4, 8, 12 mg

Indications & dosages

➤ *Mild to moderate Alzheimer's type dementia*—**Adult:** Initially, 4 mg bid, preferably with am and pm meal. If dose is well tolerated after minimum of 4 wk of therapy, increase to 8 mg bid. Attempt a further increase to 12 mg bid may be attempted only after ≥ 4 wk at previous dose. Recommended range, 16-24 mg/d in 2 divided doses.†, ‡

---

ganciclovir
Cytovene

Synthetic nucleoside; antiviral
PRC: C

Available forms

Capsules: 250, 500 mg; *Injection:* 500 mg/vial

Indications & dosages

➤ *CMV retinitis in immunocompromised patients and AIDS patients*—**Adult:** 5 mg/kg IV q 12 hr × 14-21 d; maintenance, 5 mg/kg IV daily × 7 d/wk or 6 mg/kg/d × 5 d/wk. Or, 1,000 mg PO tid with food; or, 500 mg PO q 3 hr while awake (6 times/d).†

➤ *To prevent CMV in HIV infection*—**Adult:** 1,000 mg PO tid with food.†

➤ *To prevent CMV in transplant recipients*—**Adult:** 5 mg/kg IV q 12 hr × 7-14 d, then 5 mg/kg/d × 7 d/wk; or 6 mg/kg/d × 5 d/wk.†

---

gatifloxacin (systemic)
Tequin

Fluoroquinolone; antibiotic
PRC: C

Available forms

Injection: 200 mg/20-ml vial, 400 mg/40-ml vial; 200 mg/100 ml D₅W, 400 mg/200 ml D₅W; *Tablets:* 200, 400 mg

Indications & dosages

➤ *Complicated UTI, pyelonephritis*—**Adult:** 400 mg IV or PO daily × 7-10 d.†

➤ *Sinusitis*—**Adult:** 400 mg IV or PO daily × 10 d.†
➤ *Community-acquired pneumonia*—**Adult:** 400 mg IV or PO daily × 7-14 d.†
➤ *Urethral gonorrhea in man; cervical gonorrhea or rectal infection in woman from* Neisseria gonorrhoeae—**Adult:** 400 mg PO × 1 dose.†
➤ *Uncomplicated UTI*—**Adult:** 400 mg IV or PO × 1 dose, or 200 mg IV or PO daily × 3 d.†
➤ *Acute bacterial exacerbation of chronic bronchitis from* Streptococcus pneumoniae, Haemophilus influenzae, H. parainfluenzae, Moraxella catarrhalis, *or* Staphylococcus aureus—**Adult:** 400 mg IV or PO daily × 5 d.†
➤ *Uncomplicated skin and skin-structure infections from* Staphylococcus aureus (methicillin-susceptible strains only) or Streptococcus pyogenes—**Adult:** 400 mg IV or PO daily × 7-10 d.†

gatifloxacin (ophthalmic)
Zymar

Fluoroquinolone; antibiotic
PRC: C

Available forms
Solution: 0.3% in 2.5- and 5-ml bottles

Indications & dosages
➤ *Bacterial conjunctivitis*—**Adult, child ≥ 1 yr:** While awake, instill 1 drop into affected eye q 2 hr, up to 8 times daily for 2 d. Then instill 1 drop up to qid for 5 more days.

gefitinib
Iressa

Tyrosine kinase inhibitor; antineoplastic
PRC: D

Available forms
Tablets: 250 mg

Indications & dosages
➤ *Locally advanced or metastatic non–small-cell lung CA after platinum-based and docetaxel chemo have failed*—**Adult:** 250 mg PO once daily.

gemfibrozil
Lopid

Fibric acid derivative; antilipemic
PRC: C

Available forms
Tablets: 600 mg

Indications & dosages
➤ *Types IV and V hyperlipidemia, CAD risk reduction in type IIb hyperlipidemia*—**Adult:** 1,200 mg PO daily in 2 divided doses, 30 min ac in am and pm.

gemifloxacin mesylate
Factive

Fluoroquinolone; antibiotic
PRC: C

Available forms
Tablets: 320 mg

Indications & dosages

➤ *Acute bacterial exacerbation of chronic bronchitis caused by* Streptococcus pneumoniae, Haemophilus influenzae, Haemophilus parainfluenzae, Moraxella catarrhalis—**Adult:** 320 mg PO once daily × 5 d.

➤ *Mild to moderate community-acquired pneumonia caused by* S. pneumoniae (including multi-drug–resistant strains), H. influenzae, M. catarrhalis, Mycoplasma pneumoniae, Chlamydia pneumoniae, Klebsiella pneumoniae—**Adult:** 320 mg PO once daily × 7 d.

gentamicin sulfate
Garamycin, Gentamicin Sulfate

Aminoglycoside; antibiotic
PRC: D

Available forms

Injection: 40 mg/ml (adult), 10 mg/ml (pediatric); *IV infusion (premixed):* 40, 60, 70, 80, 90, 100, 120 mg in NSS

Indications & dosages

➤ *Serious infection*—**Adult:** 3 mg/kg/d IM or IV infusion in divided doses q 8 hr. For life-threatening infection, up to 5 mg/kg/d in 3-4 divided doses; reduce to 3 mg/kg/d ASAP. **Child:** 6-7.5 mg/kg/d IM or IV infusion in divided doses q 8 hr. **Neonate > 1 wk, infant:** 7.5 mg/kg/d in divided doses q 8 hr.

➤ *To prevent endocarditis in GI, GU procedure, or surgery*—**Adult:** 1.5 mg/kg IM or IV 30 min before procedure or surgery. Max, 80 mg. **Child:** 2 mg/kg IM or IV 30 min before procedure or surgery. Max, 80 mg. After 8 hr, ½ initial dose.

glimepiride
Amaryl

Sulfonylurea; antidiabetic
PRC: C

Available forms

Tablets: 1, 2, 4 mg

Indications & dosages

➤ *Type 2 DM*—**Adult:** 1-2 mg PO daily with 1st main meal of d; maintenance, 1-4 mg PO daily. After reaching 2 mg, increase to 2 mg q 1-2 wk, based on glucose level. Max, 8 mg/d.†, ‡

➤ *Adjunct to insulin therapy in type 2 DM*—**Adult:** 8 mg PO daily with 1st main meal of d; use with low-dose insulin.†, ‡

➤ *Adjunct to metformin in type 2 DM*—**Adult:** 8 mg PO daily with 1st main meal of d with metformin. Adjust doses prn.†, ‡

glipizide
Glucotrol, Glucotrol XL

Sulfonylurea; antidiabetic
PRC: C

Available forms

Tablets: 5, 10 mg; *Tablets (extended-release):* 5, 10 mg

Indications & dosages

➤ *Type 2 DM*—**Adult:** 5 mg PO 30 min before breakfast. Maintenance 10-15 mg; max 40 mg daily. Daily doses above

§ Adjust in immunocompromised patients   ¶ Adjust in debilitated patients

15 mg can be divided bid. Or, 5 mg extended-release PO daily given with breakfast. Adjust in 5-mg increments q 3 mo. Max, 20 mg daily.‡, ¶

➤ *To replace insulin therapy*—**Adult:** If insulin dosage > 20 units daily, start at 5 mg PO daily plus 50% of insulin dose. If insulin dose < 20 units, stop insulin when starting this drug.‡, ¶

glipizide and metformin hydrochloride
Metaglip

Sulfonylurea and biguanide; antidiabetic
PRC: C

Available forms
Tablets: 2.5 mg glipizide and 250 mg metformin hydrochloride; 2.5 mg glipizide and 500 mg metformin; 5 mg glipizide and 500 mg metformin

Indications & dosages
➤ *Type 2 DM with diet and exercise*—
Adult: Initially 2.5 mg/250 mg PO daily with a meal. Patients with fasting glucose level of 280 to 320 mg/dl, start with 2.5 mg/500 mg PO bid. May increase dose by 1 tablet daily q 2 wk. Max, 10 mg/ 1,000 mg or 10 mg/2,000 mg daily in divided doses.
➤ *Type 2 DM when diet, exercise, and sulfonylurea or metformin therapy fail*—
Adult: Initially, 2.5 mg/500 mg or 5 mg/ 500 mg PO bid with am and pm meals. Increase by ≤ 5 mg/500 mg. Max, 20 mg/ 2,000 mg daily.

glucagon

Antihypoglycemic; antidiabetic, diagnostic aid
PRC: B

Available forms
Powder for injection: 1 mg (1 unit)

Indications & dosages
➤ *Hypoglycemia*—**Adult, child > 20 kg:**
1 mg SC, IM, or IV; may repeat in 15 min prn. In deep coma, also give glucose 10-50% IV. **Child ≤ 20 kg:** 0.5 mg SC, IM, or IV. In deep coma, also give glucose 10-50% IV. May repeat in 15 min prn.
➤ *Diagnostic aid for radiologic exam*—
Adult: 0.25-2 mg IV or IM before radiologic procedure.

glyburide (glibenclamide)
DiaBeta, Euglucon*, Glynase PresTab, Micronase

Sulfonylurea; antidiabetic
PRC: C

Available forms
Tablets: 1.25, 2.5, 5 mg; *Tablets (micronized):* 1.5, 3, 4.5, 6 mg

Indications & dosages
➤ *Type 2 DM*—**Adult:** 2.5-5 mg regular tablet PO daily with breakfast. Maintenance, 1.25-20 mg daily in 1 dose or divided doses or may use micronized preparation. Initially, 1.5-3 mg daily. In sensitive patients, 0.75 mg daily. Maintenance, 0.75-12 mg/d. Patients receiving > 6 mg/d, use bid. In debilitated, mal-

---

nourished, or elderly patients or those with adrenal or pituitary insufficiency, 1.25 mg/d.

➤ *To replace insulin therapy*—**Adult:** For insulin dose < 20 units/d, 2.5-5 mg/d PO and stop insulin; for 20-40 units/d, 5 mg/d PO and stop insulin; for > 40 units/d, 5 mg/d plus 50% reduction of insulin dose. Withdraw insulin gradually based on response. For micronized tablets, if insulin dose > 40 units/d, 3 mg PO with 50% reduction in insulin; if 20-40 units/d, 3 mg PO daily and stop insulin; if < 20 units/d, 1.5-3 mg/d and stop insulin. Adjust dose in malnourished or elderly patients or those with adrenal or pituitary insufficiency.¶

granisetron hydrochloride
Kytril

Selective 5-hydroxy-tryptamine receptor antagonist; antiemetic, antinauseant
PRC: B

Available forms

Injection: 1 mg/ml; *Oral solution:* 1 mg/ 5 ml; *Tablets:* 1 mg

Indications & dosages

➤ *Prevent nausea, vomiting with emetogenic CA chemo*—**Adult, child ≥ 2:** 10 mcg/kg undiluted drug IV by direct injection over 30 sec, or diluted and infused over 5 min. Start within 30 min of starting chemo. Or, for adults, 1 mg PO up to 1 hr before chemo; repeat 12 hr later. Or, for adults, 2 mg PO daily given ≤ 1 hr before chemo.

➤ *Postop nausea and vomiting*—**Adult:** 1 mg undiluted drug IV over 30 sec. For prevention, give before anesthesia induction or immediately before reversal.

➤ *To prevent nausea, vomiting with radiation*—**Adult:** 2 mg PO daily within 1 hr of radiation.

guaifenesin (glyceryl guaiacolate)
Anti-Tuss, Glytuss, Halotussin, Humibid L.A., Mucinex, Robitussin

Propanediol derivative; expectorant
PRC: C

Available forms

Capsules: 200 mg; *Capsules (sustained-release):* 300 mg; *Solution:* 100, 200 mg/ 5 ml; *Tablets:* 100, 200 mg; *Tablets (extended-release):* 600; *Tablets (sustained-release):* 575, 600, 800, 1200 mg

Indications & dosages

➤ *Expectorant*—Don't give Mucinex ER 600 mg tablets to child < 12 yr. **Adult, child ≥ 12 yr:** 100-400 mg PO q 4 hr; max 2.4 g/d. Or, 600-1,200 mg sustained- or extended-release tablets q 12 hr; max 2,400 mg/d. **Child 6-11 yr:** 100-200 mg PO q 4 hr; max, 1,200 mg/d. Or, 600 mg sustained- or extended-release tablets PO q 12 hr; max 1,200 mg/d. **Child 2-5 yr:** 50-100 mg PO q 4 hr; max 600 mg/d. Or, 300 mg sustained- or extended-release tablets q 12 hr; max 600 mg/d.

---

§ Adjust in immunocompromised patients   ¶ Adjust in debilitated patients

haloperidol
Apo-Haloperidol*, Haldol, Novo-Peridol*, Peridol*

haloperidol decanoate
Haldol Decanoate, Haldol LA*

haloperidol lactate
Haldol

Butyrophenone; antipsychotic
PRC: C

Available forms
haloperidol *Tablets:* 0.5, 1, 2, 5, 10, 20 mg; **decanoate** *Injection:* 50, 100 mg/ml; **lactate** *Injection:* 5 mg/ml; *Oral concentrate:* 2 mg/ml

Indications & dosages
➤ *Psychotic disorders*—**Adult, child ≥ 12 yr:** 0.5-5 mg PO bid or tid; or, 2-5 mg IM q 4-8 hr. Max, 100 mg PO daily. **Child 3-11 yr:** 0.05-0.15 mg/kg PO daily in 2-3 divided doses.
➤ *Chronic psychosis*—**Adult:** 50-100 mg IM decanoate q 4 wk.¶
➤ *Nonpsychotic behavior disorders*—**Child 3-12 yr:** 0.05-0.075 mg/kg PO daily in 2 or 3 divided doses. Max, 6 mg/d.

heparin sodium
Hepalean*

Anticoagulant; anticoagulant, antithrombotic
PRC: C

Available forms
sodium *Disposable syringes:* 1,000, 2,500, 5,000, 7,500, 20,000 units/ml; *Flush (disposable syringes, vials):* 10, 100 units/ml; *Premixed IV solution:* 1,000 units in 500 ml NSS; 2,000 units in 1,000 ml NSS; 12,500, 25,000 units in 250 ml ½ NSS; 25,000 units in 500 ml ½ NSS; 10,000 units in 100 ml D_5W; 12,500, 25,000 units in 250 ml D_5W; 20,000, 25,000 units in 500 ml D_5W; *Unit-dose vials:* 1,000, 5,000, 10,000, 20,000, 40,000 units/ml; *Vials:* 1,000, 2,000, 2,500, 5,000, 10,000, 20,000, 40,000 units/ml

Indications & dosages
➤ *Full-dose IV infusion therapy for DVT, MI, PE*—**Adult:** 5,000 units IV bolus; then 750-1,500 units/hr IV infusion pump. Adjust hourly rate 8 hr after bolus dose, based on PTT. **Child:** 50 units/kg IV; then 25 units/kg/hr or 20,000 units/m² daily by IV infusion pump. Adjust dose based on PTT.
➤ *Full-dose SC therapy for DVT, MI, PE*—**Adult:** 5,000 units IV bolus and 10,000-20,000 units in concentrated solution SC; then 8,000-10,000 units SC q 8 hr or 15,000-20,000 units in concentrated solution q 12 hr.
➤ *Fixed low-dose therapy for venous thrombosis, postop DVT, PE, atrial fibrillation with embolism, embolism prevention*—**Adult:** 5,000 units SC q 12 hr. In surgical patients, give 1st dose 2 hr before surgery, then 5,000 units SC q 8-12 hr × 5-7 d or until patient can walk.
➤ *Consumptive coagulopathy (such as disseminated intravascular coagula-*

tion)—**Adult:** 50-100 units/kg IV bolus or continuous IV infusion q 4 hr. **Child:** 25-50 units/kg IV bolus or continuous IV infusion q 4 hr. If no improvement within 4-8 hr, stop therapy.

hydralazine hydrochloride
Apresoline, Novo-Hylazin*

Peripheral vasodilator; antihypertensive
PRC: C

Available forms
Injection: 20 mg/ml; *Tablets:* 10, 25, 50, 100 mg

Indications & dosages
➤ *HTN (PO), severe HTN (parenteral)*—**Adult:** 10 mg PO qid; increase to 50 mg qid. Max, 200 mg/d (300-400 mg/d in some patients). Or, 10-20 mg IV repeated prn; switch to PO ASAP. Or, 20-40 mg IM repeated prn; switch to PO ASAP. **Child:** 0.75 mg/kg/d PO in 4 divided doses; increase over 3-4 wk. Max, 7.5 mg/kg or 200 mg daily. Or, 1.7-3.5 mg/kg/d or 50-100 mg/m²/d IV or IM in 4-6 divided doses. Max dose, ≤ 20 mg. If given with reserpine, decrease to 0.15 mg/kg or 4 mg/m² q 12-24 hr.

hydrochlorothiazide (HCTZ)
Apo-Hydro*, Aquazide-H, Esidrix, HydroDIURIL, Oretic

Thiazide diuretic; diuretic, antihypertensive
PRC: B

Available forms
Capsules: 12.5 mg; *Oral solution:* 50 mg/5 ml; *Tablets:* 25, 50, 100 mg

Indications & dosages
➤ *Edema*—**Adult:** 25-100 mg PO daily or intermittently.
➤ *HTN*—**Adult:** 12.5-50 mg PO daily. Increase or decrease dose based on BP. **Child 2-12 yr:** 2.2 mg/kg or 60 mg/m² daily in 2 divided doses. Usual, 37.5-100 mg/d. **Child 6 mo-2 yr:** 2.2 mg/kg or 60 mg/m² daily in 2 divided doses. Usual, 12.5-37.5 mg/d. **Child < 6 mo:** Max, 3.3 mg/kg daily in 2 divided doses.

hydrocortisone (systemic)
Cortef, Hydrocortone

hydrocortisone acetate
Cortifoam, Hydrocortone Acetate

hydrocortisone sodium phosphate
Hydrocortone Phosphate

hydrocortisone sodium succinate
A-hydroCort, Solu-Cortef

Glucocorticoid, mineralocorticoid; adrenocorticoid replacement
PRC: C

Available forms
hydrocortisone *Enema:* 100 mg/60 ml; *Tablets:* 5, 10, 20 mg; **acetate** *Enema:* 10% aerosol foam (90 mg/application); *Injection:* 25 mg/ml, 50 mg/ml suspen-

§ Adjust in immunocompromised patients   ¶ Adjust in debilitated patients

sion; **sodium phosphate** *Injection:* 50 mg/ml solution; **sodium succinate** *Injection:* 100, 250, 500, 1,000 mg/vial

Indications & dosages

➤ *Severe inflammation, adrenal insufficiency*—**Adult:** 5-30 mg PO bid-qid (up to 80 mg qid). Or, 100-500 mg succinate IM or IV, then 50-100 mg IM. Or, 15-240 mg phosphate IM or IV daily in divided doses q 12 hr; or 5-75 mg acetate into joints or soft tissue. Local anesthetics are often mixed in same syringe.

➤ *Shock*—**Adult:** 50 mg/kg succinate IV repeated in 4 hr. Repeat q 24 hr prn. Or, 100-500 mg to 2 g q 2-6 hr; continue until patient is stabilized. **Child:** 0.16-1 mg/kg phosphate (IM) or succinate (IM or IV) or 6-30 mg/m² daily or bid.

---

hydrocortisone (topical)
Acticort, CaldeCORT, Cortef, Cortizone 5

hydrocortisone acetate
CortaGel, Cortaid, Cortamed*, Hydrocortisone Acetate

hydrocortisone butyrate
Locoid

hydrocortisone valerate
Westcort

Glucocorticoid; topical adrenocorticoid
PRC: C

Available forms

hydrocortisone (topical) *Aerosol:* 0.5%, 1%; *Cream:* 0.5%, 1%, 2.5%; *Enema:* 100 mg/60 ml; *Gel:* 1%; *Lotion:* 0.25%, 0.5%, 1%, 2%, 2.5%; *Ointment:* 0.5%, 1%, 2.5%; *Pledgets:* 0.5%, 1%; *Rectal cream:* 1%; *Stick roll-on:* 1%; *Suppository:* 25 mg; *Topical solution:* 0.5%, 1%, 2.5%; **acetate** *Cream, ointment:* 0.5%, 1%; *Lotion:* 0.5%; *Paste:* 0.5%; *Rectal foam:* 90/application; *Solution:* 1%; *Suppository:* 10, 25 mg; **butyrate** *Cream, ointment, solution:* 0.1%; **valerate** *Cream, ointment:* 0.2%

Indications & dosages

➤ *Dermatitis, topical management of seborrheic scalp dermatitis*—**Adult, child:** Clean area; apply cream, gel, lotion, ointment, or topical solution sparingly once daily to qid. Spray aerosol on affected area once daily to qid for acute phase; then reduce to 1-3 times/wk prn.

➤ *Inflammation in proctitis*—**Adult:** 1 applicator rectal foam PR daily or bid × 2-3 wk; then q other d prn.

---

hydromorphone hydrochloride (dihydromorphinone hydrochloride)
Dilaudid, Dilaudid-HP

Opioid; analgesic, antitussive
PRC: C; CSS: II

Available forms

Injection: 1, 2, 4, 10 mg/ml; *Liq:* 5 mg/5 ml; *Suppository:* 3 mg; *Tablets:* 1, 2, 3, 4, 8 mg

---

Indications & dosages
➤ *Pain*—**Adult:** 2-10 mg PO q 3-6 hr prn or around-the-clock. Or, 2-4 mg IM, SC, or IV (over ≥ 3-5 min) q 4-6 hr prn or around-the-clock; or, 3 mg PR hs prn or around-the-clock. Or, give 1-14 mg Dilaudid-HP SC or IM q 4-6 hr.
➤ *Cough*—**Adult, adolescent > 12 yr:** 1 mg PO q 3-4 hr prn. **Child 6-12 yr:** 0.5 mg PO q 3-4 hr prn.

hydroxyzine hydrochloride
Apo-Hydroxyzine*, Atarax, Multipax*

hydroxyzine pamoate
Vistaril

Antihistamine (piperazine derivative); anxiolytic, sedative, antipruritic, antiemetic, antispasmodic
PRC: C

Available forms
hydrochloride *Capsules*:* 10, 25, 50 mg; *Injection:* 25, 50 mg/ml; *Syrup:* 10 mg/ 5 ml; *Tablets:* 10, 25, 50, 100 mg; **pamoate** *Capsules:* 25, 50, 100 mg; *Oral suspension:* 25 mg/5 ml

Indications & dosages
➤ *Anxiety, tension, hyperkinesias*— **Adult:** 50-100 mg PO qid. **Child ≥ 6 yr:** 50-100 mg PO daily in divided doses. **Child < 6 yr:** 50 mg PO daily in divided doses.
➤ *Preop, postop adjunctive sedation; vomiting; asthma*—**Adult:** 25-100 mg IM q 4-6 hr. **Child:** 1.1 mg/kg IM q 4-6 hr.

➤ *Pruritus from allergies*—**Adult:** 25 mg PO tid or qid. **Child ≥ 6 yr:** 50-100 mg PO daily in divided doses. **Child < 6 yr:** 50 mg PO daily in divided doses.

ibuprofen
Advil, Children's Advil, Children's Motrin, Motrin, Motrin IB, Motrin-IB Caplets, Nuprin, Nuprin Caplets, Pedia-Profen

NSAID; nonopioid analgesic, antipyretic, anti-inflammatory
PRC: B

Available forms
Tablets: 100, 200, 400, 600, 800 mg; *Tablets (chewable):* 50, 100 mg; *Oral suspension:* 100 mg/2.5 ml, 100 mg/5 ml; *Oral drops:* 40 mg/ml

Indications & dosages
➤ *RA, OA, arthritis*—**Adult:** 300-800 mg PO tid or qid. Max, 3.2 g/d.
➤ *Pain, dysmenorrhea*—**Adult:** 400 mg PO q 4-6 hr prn.
➤ *Fever*—**Adult:** 200-400 mg PO q 4-6 hr. Don't exceed 1.2 g daily or give > 3 d. **Child 6 mo-12 yr:** If temp < 39° C, 5 mg/kg PO q 6-8 hr. Higher temp, 10 mg/ kg q 6-8 hr. Max, 40 mg/kg/d.
➤ *Juvenile arthritis*—**Child:** 30-40 mg/ kg/d in 3-4 divided doses; max 50 mg/ kg/d.

---

§ Adjust in immunocompromised patients   ¶ Adjust in debilitated patients

imatinib mesylate
Gleevec

Protein-tyrosine kinase inhibitor; antineoplastic
PRC: D

Available forms
Capsules: 50, 100 mg; *Tablets:* 100, 400 mg

Indications & dosages
➤ *Philadelphia-chromosome–positive chronic myeloid leukemia (CML) in newly diagnosed patients; Philadelphia-chromosome–positive CML in blast crisis, accelerated phase, or chronic phase after failure of interferon alfa therapy*—**Adult:** For chronic-phase CML, 400 mg PO daily as single dose with a meal and large glass of H_2O. May increase dose to 600 mg PO daily.‡, § For accelerated-phase CML or blast crisis, 600 mg PO daily as single dose with a meal and large glass of H_2O. May increase to 400 mg PO bid. Continue treatment as long as patient benefits.‡, §
➤ *Kit (CD117)-positive unresectable or metastatic malignant GI stromal tumor*—**Adult:** 400 or 600 mg PO daily.‡, §

imipenem and cilastatin
Primaxin IM, Primaxin IV

Carbapenem (thienamycin class) beta-lactam antibiotic; antibiotic
PRC: C

Available forms
Powder for injection: 250, 500, 750 mg

Indications & dosages
➤ *Serious lower respiratory, urinary tract, intra-abdominal, GYN, bone, joint, skin, soft-tissue infection; bacterial septicemia and endocarditis*—**Adult, child ≥ 40 kg:** 250 mg-1 g by IV infusion q 6-8 hr. Max, 50 mg/kg/d or 4 g/d, whichever is less. Or, 500-750 mg IM q 12 hr. Don't use IM for septicemia or endocarditis. Max, 1,500 mg/d. **Child < 40 kg:** 60 mg/kg IV daily in divided doses. **Infant < 36 wk gestational age:** 20 mg/kg IV q 12 hr.†

imipramine hydrochloride
Apo-Imipramine*, Impril*, Norfranil, Tipramine, Tofranil

imipramine pamoate
Tofranil-PM

Dibenzazepine TCA; antidepressant
PRC: D

Available forms
hydrochloride *Tablets:* 10, 25, 50 mg; **pamoate** *Capsules:* 75, 100, 125, 150 mg

Indications & dosages
➤ *Depression*—**Adult:** 75-100 mg PO daily in divided doses; increase in 25-50 mg increments. Max for outpatients, 200 mg/d; inpatients, 300 mg/d. Entire dose may be given hs. **Elderly, child ≥ 12 yr:** 30-40 mg daily. Max, 100 mg/d.
➤ *Childhood enuresis*—**Child ≥ 6 yr:** 25 mg PO 1 hr before hs. If no response within 1 wk, increase to 50 mg if child < 12 yr; 75 mg if child ≥ 12 yr. Max, 2.5 mg/kg/d.

inamrinone lactate

Bipyridine derivative; inotropic, vaso-dilator
PRC: C

Available forms

Injection: 5 mg/ml

Indications & dosages

➤ *Short-term management of HF*—
Adult: Initially, 0.75 mg/kg IV bolus over 2-3 min; then begin maintenance infusion of 5-10 mcg/kg/min. Additional bolus of 0.75 mg/kg may be given 30 min after treatment starts. Max, 10 mg/kg/d.

indapamide
Lozide*, Lozol

Thiazide-like diuretic; diuretic, antihypertensive
PRC: B

Available forms

Tablets: 1.25, 2.5 mg

Indications & dosages

➤ *Edema*—**Adult:** 2.5 mg PO daily in am. Increase to 5 mg/d after 1 wk prn.
➤ *HTN*—**Adult:** 1.25 mg PO daily in am. Increase to 2.5 mg/d after 4 wk prn. Increase to 5 mg/d after 4 more wk prn.

indinavir sulfate
Crixivan

HIV protease inhibitor; antiviral
PRC: C

Available forms

Capsules: 100, 200, 333, 400 mg

Indications & dosages

➤ *HIV infection*—**Adult:** 800 mg PO q 8 hr.‡

indomethacin
Apo-Indomethacin*, Indochron ER, Indocid SR*, Indocin, Indocin SR, Novo-Methacin*

NSAID; nonopioid analgesic, antipyretic, anti-inflammatory
PRC: NR

Available forms

Capsules: 25, 50 mg; *Capsules (sustained-release):* 75 mg; *Oral suspension:* 25 mg/5 ml; *Suppository:* 50 mg

Indications & dosages

➤ *RA, OA, ankylosing spondylitis*—
Adult: 25 mg PO or PR bid or tid with food or antacids; increase daily dose 25 or 50 mg q 7 d. Max 200 mg daily. Or, 75 mg sustained-release PO in am or hs; then 75 mg bid prn.
➤ *Gouty arthritis*—**Adult:** 50 mg PO tid. Reduce ASAP; then stop.
➤ *Shoulder bursitis or tendinitis*—**Adult:** 75-150 mg PO daily in divided doses tid or qid × 7-14 d.

---

§ Adjust in immunocompromised patients   ¶ Adjust in debilitated patients

insulin injection (regular insulin, crystalline zinc insulin)
Humulin R, Iletin II Regular, Novolin R, Purified Pork

insulin (lispro)
Humalog

isophane insulin suspension (NPH)
Humulin N, Novolin N, NPH Insulin

isophane insulin suspension with insulin injection
Humulin 50/50, Humulin 70/30, Novolin 70/30

insulin zinc suspension (lente)
Humulin L, Lente Insulin

insulin zinc suspension, extended (ultralente)
Humulin U, Ultralente Insulin

insulin aspart
NovoLog

insulin glargine
Lantus

Pancreatic hormone; antidiabetic
PRC: B (C, insulin glargine and aspart)

Available forms
Injection: range 100-500 units/ml; human, pork sources; vials to cartridge systems; slow to fast acting

Indications & dosages
➤ *Moderate to severe diabetic ketoacidosis or hyperosmolar hyperglycemia*—
Adult > 20 yr: 0.15 units/kg regular insulin IV direct injection; then 0.1 units/kg/hr as continuous infusion. Decrease to 0.05-0.1 units/kg/hr when plasma glucose level 250-300 mg/dl. Start infusion of D_5W in half-NSS separately from the insulin infusion when glucose levels are 150-200 mg/dl in diabetic ketoacidosis patients or 250-300 mg/dl in hyperosmolar hyperglycemia patients. One or two hr before stopping insulin infusion, give a dose of intermediate-acting insulin SC. **Adult, child ≤ 20 yr:** Loading dose isn't recommended. Start with 0.1 units/kg/hr regular insulin IV infusion. Once condition improves, decrease to 0.05 units/kg/hr. Start infusion of D_5W in half-NSS separately from the insulin infusion when glucose level is 250 mg/dl.
➤ *Mild diabetic ketoacidosis*—**Adult > 20 yr:** Loading dose of 0.4-0.6 units/kg regular insulin divided equally in 2 parts with ½ the dose given by direct IV injection and the other ½ given IM or SC. Subsequent doses can be based on 0.1 units/kg/hr IM or SC.
➤ *Newly diagnosed DM*—**Adult > 20 yr:** Individualize therapy. Initially, 0.5-1 units/kg/d regular insulin SC as part of a regimen with short- and long-acting insulin therapy. **Adult, child ≤ 20 yr:** Individualize

therapy. Initially, 0.1-0.25 units/kg regular insulin SC q 6 to 8 hr × 24 hr, then adjust accordingly.

➤ *Control of hyperglycemia in patients with type 1 DM*—**Adult:** Dosage varies among patients and must be determined by a health care professional familiar with patient's metabolic needs, eating habits, and other lifestyle variables. Inject with Humalog and longer-acting insulin SC within 15 min ac or immediately pc.

➤ *Control of hyperglycemia in patients with type 2DM*—**Adult, child > 3 yr:** Dosage varies among patients and must be determined by a health care professional familiar with patient's metabolic needs, eating habits, and other lifestyle variables. Inject Humalog and sulfonylureas SC within 15 min ac or immediately pc.

ipratropium bromide
Atrovent

Anticholinergic; bronchodilator
PRC: B

Available forms

Inhalation: 18 mcg/metered dose; *Nasal spray:* 0.03% (21 mcg/metered dose), 0.06% (42 mcg/metered dose); *Solution (for inhalation):* 0.02% (500 mcg/vial)

Indications & dosages

➤ *Bronchospasm in COPD*—**Adult, child > 12 yr:** 1 or 2 inhalations qid. Max, 12 inhalations/24 hr. Or, inhalation solution 500 mcg dissolved in NSS via nebulizer q 6-8 hr.

➤ *Rhinorrhea from allergic and nonallergic perennial rhinitis*—**Adult, child ≥ 6 yr:** 2 sprays 0.3% nasal spray (42 mcg) per nostril bid or tid.

➤ *Rhinorrhea from common cold*—**Adult, child ≥ 12 yr:** 2 sprays 0.6% nasal spray (84 mcg) per nostril tid or qid. **Child 5-11 yr:** 2 sprays 0.6% nasal spray (84 mcg) per nostril tid.

➤ *Rhinorrhea associated with seasonal allergic rhinitis*—**Adult, child ≥ 5 yr:** 2 sprays 0.06% nasal spray (84 mcg) per nostril qid.

irbesartan
Avapro

Angiotensin II receptor antagonist; antihypertensive
PRC: C (D, 2nd and 3rd trimesters)

Available forms

Tablet: 75, 150, 300 mg

Indications & dosages

➤ *HTN*—**Adult, child ≥ 13 yr:** 150 mg PO daily; increase to max 300 mg daily prn. Decrease dose in volume- and salt-depleted patients. **Child 6-12 yr:** 75 mg PO daily; increase to max 150 mg daily prn.

➤ *Nephropathy in type 2 DM*—**Adult:** 300 mg PO daily.

isoniazid (isonicotinic acid hydrazide, INH)

Isotamine*, Laniazid, Nydrazid, PMS-Isoniazid*

Isonicotinic acid hydrazine; antituberculotic
PRC: C

Available forms

Injection: 100 mg/ml; *Oral solution:* 50 mg/5 ml; *Tablets:* 100, 300 mg

Indications & dosages

➤ *Active tubercle bacilli*—**Adult:** 5-10 mg/kg PO or IM daily. Max, 300 mg/d × 9 mo-2 yr. **Infant, child:** 10-20 mg/kg PO or IM daily. Max, 300 mg/d × 18 mo-2 yr. Give with 1 other antituberculotic.
➤ *Prevent tubercle bacilli in patients exposed to TB or with nonprogressive TB*—**Adult:** 300 mg PO daily in 1 dose, continue × 6 mo. **Infant, child:** 10 mg/kg PO daily in 1 dose. Max, 300 mg/d; continue × 6 mo.

isoproterenol hydrochloride

Isuprel

Adrenergic; bronchodilator, cardiac stimulant
PRC: C

Available forms

Injection: 20, 200 mcg/ml

Indications & dosages

➤ *Shock*—**Adult, child:** 0.5-5 mcg/min by continuous IV infusion titrated prn.

➤ *Bronchospasm during anesthesia*—**Adult:** 0.01-0.02 mg IV. Repeat prn.
➤ *Heart block, ventricular arrhythmias*—**Adult:** 0.02-0.06 mg IV; then 0.01-0.2 mg IV or 5 mcg/min IV, titrated prn. Or, 0.2 mg IM; then 0.02-1 mg IM prn. **Child:** IV infusion 2.5 mcg/min or 0.1 mcg/kg/min. Titrate prn.

isosorbide dinitrate

Apo-ISDN*, Dilatrate-SR, Isonate, Isorbid, Isordil, Isordil Tembids, Isotrate, Sorbitrate

isosorbide mononitrate

Imdur, ISMO, Monoket

Nitrate; antianginal, vasodilator
PRC: C

Available forms

dinitrate *Capsules (sustained-release):* 40 mg; *Tablets:* 5, 10, 20, 30, 40 mg; *Tablets (chewable):* 5, 10 mg; *Tablets (SL):* 2.5, 5, 10 mg; *Tablets (sustained-release):* 40 mg; **mononitrate** *Tablets:* 10, 20 mg; *Tablets (extended-release):* 30, 60, 120 mg

Indications & dosages

➤ *Angina; to prevent angina attacks*—**Adult:** 2.5-10 mg SL; repeat q 5-10 min (max, 3 doses/30 min). Prevention, 2.5-10 mg SL q 2-3 hr. Or, for acute attack, 5-10 mg chewable tablets prn; for prevention, q 2-3 hr (after initial test dose of 5 mg). Or, for prevention, 5-30 mg dinitrate PO tid or qid; 20-40 mg PO sustained-release q 6-12 hr. Or, 30-60 mg Imdur PO daily on arising; increase to

120 mg daily after several d prn. Or, 20 mg ISMO or Monoket PO bid, given 7 hr apart.

itraconazole
Sporanox

Synthetic triazole; antifungal
PRC: C

Available forms
Capsules: 100 mg; *Injection:* 10 mg/ml; *Oral solution:* 10 mg/ml

Indications & dosages
➤ *Pulmonary, extrapulmonary blastomycosis; nonmeningeal histoplasmosis*—**Adult:** 200 mg PO daily. Increase dose prn in 100-mg increments. Max, 400 mg daily. Give doses > 200 mg daily in 2 divided doses. Or, 200 mg IV over 1 hr bid in 4 doses, then 200 mg IV daily. Max, 14 d. †
➤ *Aspergillosis*—**Adult:** 200-400 mg PO daily. Or, 200 mg IV over 1 hr bid in 4 doses, then 200 mg IV daily. Max, 14 d. †
➤ *Oropharyngeal, esophageal candidiasis*—**Adult:** 200 mg swished in mouth for several sec, then swallowed, daily × 7 to 14 d.

ketoconazole (oral)
Nizoral

Imidazole derivative; antifungal
PRC: C

Available forms
Tablets: 200 mg

Indications & dosages
➤ *Fungal infection*—**Adult:** 200 mg PO daily. Max, 400 mg/d. **Child ≥ 2 yr:** 3.3-6.6 mg/kg PO daily.

ketoconazole (topical)
Nizoral, Nizoral A-D

Imidazole derivative; antifungal
PRC: C

Available forms
Cream: 2%; *Shampoo:* 1%, 2%

Indications & dosages
➤ *Tinea corporis, seborrheic dermatitis, cutaneous candidiasis*—**Adult:** Cover affected and surrounding area with cream daily ≥ 2 wk; for seborrheic dermatitis, apply bid × 4 wk. Shampoo 2 times/wk × 4 wk, with ≥ 3 d between shampoos prn.
➤ *Tinea infestations*—**Adult, child:** Apply daily or bid × 2 wk; tinea pedis, × 4 wk.

ketoprofen
Orudis, Orudis KT, Oruvail

NSAID; nonopioid analgesic, antipyretic, anti-inflammatory
PRC: B

Available forms
Capsules: 25, 50, 75 mg; *Capsules (extended-release):* 100, 150, 200 mg; *Tablets:* 12.5 mg

---

§ Adjust in immunocompromised patients   ¶ Adjust in debilitated patients

Indications & dosages
➤ *RA, OA*—**Adult:** 75 mg tid. Or, 50 mg qid or 150-200 mg extended-release daily. Max, 300 mg/d.
➤ *Pain, dysmenorrhea*—**Adult:** 25-50 mg PO q 6-8 hr prn.
➤ *Minor aches, pain, fever*—**Adult:** 12.5 mg q 4-6 hr. Max, 75 mg/24 hr.

ketorolac tromethamine (systemic)
Toradol

NSAID; analgesic
PRC: C

Available forms
Injection: 15, 30 mg/ml; *Tablets:* 10 mg

Indications & dosages
➤ *Pain*—**Adult < 65 yr:** 60 mg IM or 30 mg IV in 1 dose, or multiple doses of 30 mg IM or IV q 6 hr. Max,120 mg/d.
Elderly ≥ 65 yr: 30 mg IM or 15 mg IV in 1 dose, or multiple doses of 15 mg IM or IV q 6 hr. Max, 60 mg daily. Adjust dose in patients < 50 kg.†
➤ *To switch from parenteral to PO therapy*—**Adult < 65 yr:** 20 mg PO in 1 dose; then 10 mg PO q 4-6 hr. Max, 40 mg/d.
Elderly ≥ 65 yr or those < 50 kg: 10 mg PO in 1 dose; then 10 mg PO q 4-6 hr. Max, 40 mg/d.†

labetalol hydrochloride
Normodyne, Trandate

Alpha and beta blocker; antihypertensive
PRC: C

Available forms
Injection: 5 mg/ml; *Tablets:* 100, 200, 300 mg

Indications & dosages
➤ *HTN*—**Adult:** 100 mg PO bid with or without diuretic. May increase by 100 mg bid daily q 2-4 d prn.
Maintenance, 200-600 mg bid. Max, 2,400 mg/d.
➤ *HTN emergencies*—**Adult:** Infuse 0.5-2 mg/min and titrate; usual cumulative dose, 50-200 mg. Or, 20 mg repeated IV injection over 2 min. Repeat injection of 40-80 mg q 10 min to max 300 mg.

lactulose
Cephulac, Cholac, Chronulac, Constilac, Constulose, Duphalac, Enulose, PMS-Lactulose*

Disaccharide; laxative
PRC: B

Available forms
Crystals for reconstitution: 10, 20 g/packet; *Solution (PO, PR):* 3.33 g/5 ml; *Syrup (PO):* 10 g/15 ml

Indications & dosages
➤ *Constipation*—**Adult:** 10-20 g (15-30 ml) PO daily, increase to 40 g/d prn.
➤ *Hepatic encephalopathy*—**Adult:** 20-30 g PO tid or qid until 2-3 soft BM daily.

Or, 300 ml diluted with 700 ml H$_2$O or NSS PR and retained × 40-60 min q 4-6 hr prn.

lamivudine
Epivir, Epivir-HBV

Synthetic nucleoside analogue; antiviral
PRC: C

Available forms
Oral solution: 10 mg/ml; *Tablets:* 100, 150, 300 mg

Indications & dosages
➤ *HIV infection*—**Adult, child ≥ 16 yr:** 300 mg PO daily or 150 mg PO bid. Give with other antiretrovirals.† **Child 3 mo-16 yr:** 4 mg/kg PO bid. Max, 150 mg bid. Give with other antiretrovirals.†
➤ *Chronic HBV infection given with other antiretrovirals*—**Adult:** 100 mg PO daily.† **Child 2-17 yr:** 3 mg/kg PO daily; max 100 mg daily.†

lamivudine and zidovudine
Combivir

Synthetic nucleoside analogue; antiviral
PRC: C

Available forms
Tablets: 150 mg lamivudine and 300 mg zidovudine

Indications & dosages
➤ *HIV infection*—**Adult, child ≥ 12 yr or > 50 kg:** 1 tablet PO bid.

lamotrigine
Lamictal

Phenyltriazine; anticonvulsant
PRC: C

Available forms
Tablets: 25, 100, 150, 200 mg; *Tablets (chewable dispersible):* 2, 5, 25 mg

Indications & dosages
➤ *Partial seizures*—**Adult, child > 12 yr:** 50 mg PO daily × 2 wk; then 100 mg/d in 2 divided doses × 2 wk. Maintenance, 300-500 mg PO daily in 2 divided doses. For patients also taking valproic acid, 25 mg PO q other d × 2 wk; then 25 mg PO daily × 2 wk. Max, 75 mg PO bid.†

lansoprazole
Prevacid, Prevacid SoluTab

Acid proton pump inhibitor; antiulcerative
PRC: B

Available forms
Capsules (delayed-release): 15, 30 mg; *Oral suspension (delayed-release):* 15, 30 mg/packet; *Orally disintegrating tablets (extended-release):* 15, 30 mg

Indications & dosages
➤ *Active duodenal ulcer*—**Adult:** 15 mg PO daily ac × 4 wk.
➤ *Erosive esophagitis*—**Adult:** 30 mg PO daily ac ≤ 8 wk; may give × 8 more wk prn. Maintenance, 15 mg PO daily; safety and effectiveness not established for therapy over 1 yr.

---

§ Adjust in immunocompromised patients   ¶ Adjust in debilitated patients

➤ Hypersecretory conditions, including Zollinger-Ellison syndrome—**Adult:** 60 mg PO daily. Increase dose prn. Give daily doses > 120 mg in divided doses.

➤ Reduce risk of NSAID-related ulcer in patients with history of gastric ulcer and need for NSAIDs—**Adult:** 15 mg PO daily × ≤ 12 wk.

➤ NSAID-related ulcer in patients who continue to take NSAIDs—**Adult:** 30 mg PO daily × 8 wk.

➤ Short-term therapy for symptomatic GERD and erosive esophagitis—**Child 1-11 yr ≤ 30 kg:** 15 mg PO daily for ≤ 12 wk. **Child 1-11 yr > 30 kg:** 30 mg PO daily for ≤ 12 wk.

latanoprost
Xalatan

Prostaglandin analogue; antiglaucoma drug, ocular antihypertensive
PRC: C

Available forms
Ophthalmic solution: 0.005% (50 mcg/ml)

Indications & dosages
➤ First-line therapy for increased IOP in patients with ocular HTN or open-angle glaucoma—**Adult:** 1 drop in conjunctival sac of affected eye q pm.

leflunomide
Arava

Pyrimidine synthesis inhibitor; anti-proliferative, anti-inflammatory
PRC: X

Available forms
Tablets: 10, 20, 100 mg

Indications & dosages
➤ RA—**Adult:** 100 mg PO q 24 hr × 3 d; then 20 mg (max daily dose) PO q 24 hr. Reduce dose to 10 mg/d if not well tolerated.‡

leucovorin calcium (citrovorum factor, folinic acid)

Formyl derivative (active reduced form of folic acid); vitamin, antidote
PRC: C

Available forms
Injection: 1-ml ampule (3 mg/ml with 0.9% benzyl alcohol; 10 mg/ml in 5-ml vial; 50-mg, 100-mg, and 350-mg vials for reconstitution (contain no preservatives); Tablets: 5, 15, 25 mg

Indications & dosages
➤ Folic acid–antagonist overdose—**Adult, child:** IM or IV dose equivalent to wt of antagonist.

➤ Leucovorin rescue after high methotrexate dose—**Adult, child:** 10 mg/m² PO, IM, or IV q 6 hr until methotrexate level < 5 × 10⁻⁸ M.

➤ Megaloblastic anemia from congenital enzyme deficiency—**Adult, child:** 3-6 mg IM daily.

➤ Folate-deficient megaloblastic anemia—**Adult, child:** ≤ 1 mg IM daily.

levetiracetam
Keppra

Antiepileptic; anticonvulsant
PRC: C

Available forms
Tablets: 250, 500, 750 mg; *Oral solution:* 100 mg/ml

Indications & dosages
➤ *Partial onset seizures*—**Adult:** 500 mg PO bid. Increase by 500 mg PO bid q 2 wk prn; max, 1,500 mg PO bid.†

levodopa
Dopar, Larodopa

Dopamine precursor; antiparkinsonian
PRC: C

Available forms
Capsules: 100, 250, 500 mg; *Tablets:* 100, 250, 500 mg

Indications & dosages
➤ *Parkinsonism*—**Adult:** 0.5-1 g PO daily divided bid, tid, or qid with food; increase by 100-750 mg q 3-7 d; usual dose 3-6 g daily divided into 3 doses. Max, 8 g/d except in rare patients.

levodopa and carbidopa
Sinemet, Sinemet CR

Decarboxylase inhibitor, dopamine precursor; antiparkinsonian
PRC: C

Available forms
Tablets: carbidopa 10 mg and levodopa 100 mg (Sinemet 10-100), carbidopa 25 mg and levodopa 100 mg (Sinemet 25-100), carbidopa 25 mg and levodopa 250 mg (Sinemet 25-250); *Tablets (extended-release):* carbidopa 50 mg and levodopa 200 mg, carbidopa 25 mg and levodopa 100 mg (Sinemet CR)

Indications & dosages
➤ *Parkinson's disease, symptomatic parkinsonism*—**Adult:** 1 tablet of 25 mg carbidopa and 100 mg levodopa PO tid; increase by 1 tablet daily or q other d prn, to max 8 tablets daily (25 mg carbidopa and 250 mg levodopa or 10 mg carbidopa and 100 mg levodopa tablet substituted prn, for max response). For extended-release, dose calculated on current levodopa intake. Initially, dose should amount to 10% more levodopa per d; increase prn to 30% more per d in divided doses q 4-8 hr.

levodopa, carbidopa, and entacapone
Stalevo

Dopamine precursor, decarboxylase, and COMT inhibitor; antiparkinsonian
PRC: C

Available forms
Tablets (film-coated): 50 mg levodopa, 12.5 mg carbidopa, 200 mg entacapone; 100 mg levodopa, 25 mg carbidopa, 200 mg entacapone; 150 mg levodopa, 37.5 mg carbidopa, 200 mg entacapone

---

§ Adjust in immunocompromised patients   ¶ Adjust in debilitated patients

Indications & dosages
➤ *Parkinson's disease*—**Adult:** 1 tablet PO with dose and interval determined by therapeutic response. Max, 8 tablets daily.

levofloxacin
Levaquin

Fluoroquinolone; antibiotic
PRC: C

Available forms
Single-use vials: 500 mg; *Infusion (pre-mixed in D₅W):* 250 mg/50 ml, 500 mg/100 ml, 750 mg/150 ml; *Tablets:* 250, 500, 750 mg

Indications & dosages
➤ *Maxillary sinusitis*—**Adult:** 500 mg PO or IV daily × 10-14 d.†
➤ *Exacerbation of chronic bronchitis*—**Adult:** 500 mg PO or IV daily × 7 d.†
➤ *Complicated skin infection*—**Adult:** 750 mg PO or IV q 24 hr × 7-14 d.†
➤ *Uncomplicated UTI*—**Adult:** 250 mg PO daily × 3 d.†
➤ *Uncomplicated skin infection*—**Adult:** 500 mg PO or IV daily × 7-10 d.†
➤ *Complicated UTI, acute pyelonephritis*—**Adult:** 250 mg PO or IV q 24 h × 10 d.†
➤ *Community-acquired pneumonia from PCN-resistant Streptococcus pneumoniae*—**Adult:** 500 mg PO or IV infusion over 60 min once daily × 7-14 d.†
➤ *Community-acquired pneumonia from PCN-susceptible Streptococcus pneumoniae, Haemophilus influenzae, Haemophilus parainfluenzae, Mycoplasma pneumo-*

niae, *or Chlamydia pneumoniae*—**Adult:** 750 mg PO or IV daily × 5 d.†
➤ *Nosocomial pneumonia*—**Adult:** 750 mg PO or IV daily × 7-14 d.†
➤ *Chronic bacterial prostatitis*—**Adult:** 500 mg PO or IV daily × 28 d.†

levothyroxine sodium (T₄ or L-thyroxine sodium)
Eltroxin*, Levo-T, Levothroid, Levoxine, Levoxyl, Novothyrox, Synthroid, Thyro-Tabs, Unithroid

Thyroid hormone; thyroid hormone replacement
PRC: A

Available forms
Injection: 200, 500 mcg/vial; *Tablets:* 25, 50, 75, 88, 100, 112, 125, 137, 150, 175, 200, 300 mcg

Indications & dosages
➤ *Myxedema coma*—**Adult:** 200-500 mcg IV; if no response in 24 hr, 100-300 mcg IV. Maintenance, 50-200 mcg IV daily.
➤ *Thyroid hormone replacement*—**Adult < 50 yr or adult > 50 yr recently treated for hyperthyroidism or who has been hypothyroid for short time:** Initially, 1.7 mcg/kg/d PO. **Adult > 50 yr or adult < 50 yr with underlying CV disease:** 25-50 mcg PO daily. May increase at intervals of 6-8 wk. **Elderly with underlying CV disease:** 12.5 -25 mcg PO daily. May increase by 12.5-25 mcg increments every 4-6 wk. **Adults with severe, long-standing hypothyroidism:** 12.5 mcg PO daily. May increase by 25 mcg increments every

4-8 wk. **Child > 12 yr (growth and puberty complete):** 1.6-1.7 mcg/kg/d. **Child > 12 yr (growth and puberty incomplete):** 2-3 mcg/kg/d. **Child 6-12 yr:** 4-5 mcg/kg/d. **Child 1-5 yr:** 5-6 mcg/kg/d. **Child 6-12 mo:** 6-8 mcg/kg/d. **Child 3-6 mo:** 8-10 mcg/kg/d. **Child 0-3 mo:** 10-15 mcg/kg/d.

lidocaine hydrochloride (lignocaine hydrochloride)
LidoPen Auto-Injector, Xylocaine

Amide derivative; ventricular antiarrhythmic, local anesthetic
PRC: B

Available forms
Infusion (premixed): 0.2% (2 mg/ml), 0.4% (4 mg/ml), 0.8% (8 mg/ml); *Injection (IM):* 300 mg/3 ml automatic injection device; *Injection (direct IV):* 1% (10 mg/ml), 2% (20 mg/ml); *Injection (IV admixtures):* 4% (40 mg/ml), 10% (100 mg/ml), 20% (200 mg/ml)

Indications & dosages
➤ *Ventricular arrhythmias*—**Adult:** 50-100 mg (1-1.5 mg/kg) IV bolus at 25-50 mg/min. Repeat bolus dose q 5-10 min prn or as tolerated. Max 300-mg total bolus over 1 hr. At same time, begin infusion of 20-50 mcg/kg/min (1-4 mg/min). **Elderly:** Reduce dose and rate of infusion by 50%. **Child:** 0.5-1 mg/kg IV bolus; then infusion of 10-50 mcg/kg/min. For advanced cardiac life support in children: 1 mg/kg by IV or intraosseous infusion followed by maintenance infusion of 20-

50 mcg/kg/min if necessary. Adjust dose in patients < 50 kg or with HF. ‡, †

linezolid
Zyvox

Oxazolidinone; antibiotic
PRC: C

Available forms
Injection: 2 mg/ml; *Powder for oral suspension:* 100 mg/5 ml (reconstituted); *Tablets:* 400, 600 mg

Indications & dosages
➤ *Vancomycin-resistant* Enterococcus faecium *infections, including those with concurrent bacteremia*—**Adult, child ≥ 12 yr:** 600 mg IV or PO q 12 hr × 14-28 d. **Neonate ≥ 7 d, infant, child < 12 yr:** 10 mg/kg IV or PO q 8 hr × 14-28 d. **Neonate < 7 d:** 10 mg/kg IV or PO q 12 hr. Increase to 10 mg/kg q 8 hr when patient is 7 d old or doesn't fully respond.
➤ *Nosocomial pneumonia caused by* Staphylococcus aureus *(methicillin-susceptible [MSSA] and methicillin-resistant [MRSA]) or* Streptococcus pneumonia *(penicillin-susceptible strains only); complicated skin and skin-structure infections including diabetic foot infections without osteomyelitis caused by* S. aureus *(MSSA & MRSA),* Streptococcus pyogenes, *or* Streptococcus agalactiae; *community-acquired pneumonia caused by* S. pneumoniae, *including those with concurrent bacteremia, or* S. aureus *(MSSA only)*—**Adult, child ≥ 12 yr:** 600 mg IV or PO q 12 hr × 10-14 d. **Neonate ≥ 7 d, infant, child < 12 yr:**

10 mg/kg IV or PO q 8 hr × 10-14 d.
Neonate < 7 d: 10 mg/kg IV or PO q
12 hr. Increase to 10 mg/kg q 8 hr when
patient is 7 d old or doesn't fully respond.
➤ *Uncomplicated skin and skin-
structure infections from Staphylococcus
aureus (MSSA only) or Streptococcus
pyogenes*—**Adult:** 400 mg PO q 12 hr ×
10-14 d. **Child 12-18 yr:** 600 mg PO q
12 hr × 10-14 d. **Child 5-11 yr:** 10 mg/kg
PO q 12 hr × 10-14 d. **Neonate ≥ 7 d, infant, child < 5 yr:** 10 mg/kg PO q 8 hr ×
10-14 d. **Neonate < 7 d:** 10 mg/kg IV or
PO q 12 hr. Increase to 10 mg/kg q 8 hr
when patient is 7 d old or doesn't fully
respond.

lisinopril
Prinivil, Zestril

ACE inhibitor; antihypertensive
PRC: C (D, 2nd and 3rd trimesters)

Available forms
Tablets: 2.5, 5, 10, 20, 40 mg

Indications & dosages
➤ *HTN*—**Adult:** Initially, 5-10 mg PO
daily. Usual range, 20-40 mg daily. Start
patients taking diuretics on 5 mg daily.
Child 6-16 yr: Initially 0.07 mg/kg PO
once daily (up to 5 mg total).
➤ *HF*—**Adult:** Initially, 5 mg PO daily with
diuretics and cardiac glycosides. Usual
range, 5-20 mg/d.
➤ *Acute MI*—**Adult:** 5 mg PO; then 5 mg
in 24 hr, 10 mg in 48 hr; then 10 mg/d ×
6 wk. In patients with systolic BP ≤ 120
when treatment begins or during first 3 d
after MI, reduce to 2.5 mg PO. If systolic

BP ≤ 100, reduce maintenance dose from
5 to 2.5 mg/d.

lithium carbonate
Carbolith*, Eskalith CR, Lithobid,
Lithonate, Lithotabs

lithium citrate
Cibalith-S

Alkali metal; antimanic, antipsychotic
PRC: D

Available forms
5 ml lithium citrate contains 8 mEq lithium = 300 mg lithium carbonate
carbonate *Capsules:* 150, 300, 600 mg;
Tablets: 300 mg (300 mg = 8.12 mEq
lithium); *Tablets (controlled-release):* 300,
450 mg; **citrate** *Syrup (sugarless):* 8 mEq
(lithium)/5 ml

Indications & dosages
➤ *Mania*—**Adult:** 300-600 mg PO up to
qid, or 900 mg Eskalith CR PO q 12 hr;
increase based on drug level prn.

loperamide
Imodium A-D, Kaopectate II Caplets

Piperidine derivative; antidiarrheal
PRC: B

Available forms
Capsules, caplets: 2 mg; *Oral liq:* 1 mg/
5 ml

Indications & dosages
➤ *Diarrhea*—**Adult, child ≥ 12 yr:** 4 mg
PO; then 2 mg after each unformed BM.

Max, 16 mg daily. **Child 9-11 yr:** 2 mg PO tid, d 1. **Child 6-8 yr:** 2 mg PO bid, d 1. **Child 2-5 yr:** 1 mg PO tid, d 1. Maintenance, ⅓ to ½ initial dose for child < 11 yr.

lopinavir and ritonavir
Kaletra

Protease inhibitor; antiviral
PRC: C

Available forms

Capsules: lopinavir 133.3 mg and ritonavir 33.3 mg; *Solution:* lopinavir 400 mg and ritonavir 100 mg/5 ml (80 mg/20 mg per ml)

Indications & dosages

➤ *HIV infection (with other antiretrovirals)*—**Adult, child > 12 yr:** 400 mg lopinavir and 100 mg ritonavir (3 capsules or 5 ml) PO bid with food. If susceptibility to lopinavir is suspected, consider dose of 533 mg and 133 mg (4 capsules or 6.5 ml) PO bid with food. **Child 6 mo-12 yr and 15-40 kg:** 10 mg/kg (lopinavir content) PO bid with food; max 400/100 mg in child > 40 kg. If reduced susceptibility to lopinavir is suspected, may give dose of 11 mg/kg (lopinavir content) PO bid. Treatment-experienced child > 50 kg can receive adult dose. **Child 6 mo-12 yr and 7 to < 15 kg:** 12 mg/kg (lopinavir content) PO bid with food. If reduced susceptibility to lopinavir is suspected, may give dose of 13 mg/kg (lopinavir content) PO bid with food.

loratadine
Alavert, Claritin

Tricyclic antihistamine; antihistaminic
PRC: B

Available forms

Syrup: 1 mg/ml; *Tablets:* 10 mg; *Tablets (rapidly disintegrating):* 10 mg

Indications & dosages

➤ *Seasonal allergic rhinitis, urticaria*—**Adult, child ≥ 6 yr:** 10 mg PO daily.‡, †
Child 2-5 yr: 5 mg PO daily.

lorazepam
Alzapam, Apo-Lorazepam*, Ativan, Lorazepam Intensol, Novo-Lorazem*, Nu-Loraz*

Benzodiazepine; anxiolytic, sedative-hypnotic
PRC: D; CSS: IV

Available forms

Injection: 2, 4 mg/ml; *Oral solution (concentrate):* 2 mg/ml; *Tablets:* 0.5, 1, 2 mg; *Tablets (SL):* 0.5*, 1*, 2 mg

Indications & dosages

➤ *Anxiety, agitation, irritability*—**Adult:** 2-6 mg PO daily in divided doses. Max 10 mg daily. Or, 0.05 mg/kg up to 4 mg IM daily in divided doses, or 0.044-0.05 mg/kg up to 4 mg IV daily in divided doses.
➤ *Insomnia*—**Adult:** 2-4 mg PO hs.
➤ *Preop sedation*—**Adult:** 0.05 mg/kg IM 2 hr preop. Max, 4 mg. Or, 0.044 mg/kg,

---

§ Adjust in immunocompromised patients   ¶ Adjust in debilitated patients

max, 2 mg IV, 15-20 min preop. **Adult <
50 yr:** May give 0.05 mg/kg; max, 4 mg.

losartan potassium
Cozaar

*Angiotensin II receptor antagonist; anti-
hypertensive*
PRC: C (D, 2nd and 3rd trimesters)

Available forms
Tablets: 25, 50, 100 mg

Indications & dosages
➤ *HTN*—**Adult:** 25-50 mg PO daily. Max,
100 mg daily in 1 dose or divided bid. Ad-
just dose in patients with intravascular
volume depletion.‡
➤ *Nephropathy in type 2 DM*—**Adult:**
50 mg PO daily. Increase to 100 mg daily
based on BP response.
➤ *Reduce risk of stroke in patients with
HTN and left ventricular hypertrophy*—
Adult: 50 mg PO daily; adjust based on
BP and add hydrochlorothiazide 12.5 mg
PO daily.

lovastatin (mevinolin)
Altocor, Mevacor

HMG-CoA reductase inhibitor; antilipemic
PRC: X

Available forms
Tablets: 10, 20, 40 mg; *Tablets (extended-
release):* 10, 20, 40, 60 mg

Indications & dosages
➤ *Primary prevention and treatment of
CAD; hyperlipidemia*—**Adult:** 20 mg PO

daily with pm meal. Dose range 10-80 mg
daily or divided bid. Or, 20-60 mg
extended-release PO hs. Starting dose of
10 mg can be used for patients requiring
smaller reductions. For patients also taking cyclosporine, 10 mg PO daily. Max,
20 mg daily. Don't exceed 20 mg daily in
patients also taking fibrates or niacin.†
➤ *Heterozygous familial hypercholesterolemia*—**Child 10-17 yr (girls should be
≥ 1 yr postmenarche):** 10-40 mg/d PO
with pm meal. Patients requiring ≥ 20%
reduction in LDL level, start with 20 mg/d.

magnesium chloride
Slow-Mag

magnesium sulfate

*Mineral, electrolyte; nutritional supple-
ment*
PRC: NR

Available forms
chloride *Injection:* 20% in 50-ml vial;
Tablets (delayed-release): 64 mg; **sulfate**
Injection solution: 10, 12.5, 50% in 2-, 5-,
10-, 20-, 30-, 50-ml ampules, vials, prefilled syringes

Indications & dosages
➤ *Hypomagnesemia*—**Adult:** 1 g of 50%
solution IM q 6 hr × 4 doses, depending
on magnesium level. Or, 3 g PO q 6 hr ×
4 doses.
➤ *Severe symptomatic hypomagnesemia
(magnesium level ≤ 0.8 mEq/L)*—**Adult:**
5 g IV in 1 L solution over 3 hr, then
reevaluate.

---

*Canadian   †Adjust in renal impairment   ‡ Adjust in liver impairment

➤ *Magnesium supplementation*—**Adult:** 2 tablets PO daily, or up to 2 mEq/kg IM within 4 hr prn. As part of total parenteral nutrition, 5-8 mEq daily.

magnesium citrate (citrate of magnesia)
Citroma, Citro-Mag*, Citro-Nesia, Evac-Q-Mag

magnesium hydroxide (milk of magnesia)
Milk of Magnesia, Phillips' Chewable, Phillips' Milk of Magnesia

magnesium sulfate (Epsom salts)

Magnesium salt; antacid, antiulcerative, laxative
PRC: NR

Available forms
citrate *Oral solution:* About 1.75 g magnesium/30 ml; **hydroxide** *Oral suspension:* 400, 800 mg/5 ml; *Tablets (chewable):* 311 mg; **sulfate** *Granules:* About 40 mEq magnesium/5 g

Indications & dosages
➤ *Constipation, bowel evacuation*—All doses may be single or divided. **Adult, child ≥ 12 yr:** 11-25 g citrate PO daily; 2.4-4.8 g (30-60 ml) hydroxide PO daily; 10-30 g sulfate PO daily. **Child 6-12 yr:** 5.5-12.5 g citrate PO daily; 1.2-2.4 g (15-30 ml) hydroxide PO daily; 5-10 g sulfate PO daily. **Child 2-6 yr:** 2.7-6.25 g citrate PO daily; 0.4-1.2 g (5-15 ml) hydroxide PO daily; 2.5-5 g sulfate PO daily.

➤ *Antacid*—**Adult, child > 12 yr:** 5-15 ml hydroxide suspension PO up to qid, or 622-1,244 mg hydroxide tablets PO up to qid.

magnesium oxide
Mag-Ox 400, Maox 420, Uro-Mag

Magnesium salt; antacid, laxative
PRC: NR

Available forms
Capsules: 140 mg; *Tablets:* 400, 420 mg

Indications & dosages
➤ *Antacid*—**Adult:** 140 mg PO with H_2O or milk pc and hs.
➤ *Laxative*—**Adult:** 4 g PO with H_2O or milk, usually hs.
➤ *Hypomagnesemia*—**Adult:** 400-840 mg PO daily.

magnesium sulfate

Mineral, electrolyte; anticonvulsant
PRC: A

Available forms
Injection: 4, 8, 10, 12.5, 25, 50%; *Injection solution:* 1, 2% in D_5W

Indications & dosages
➤ *Seizures in preeclampsia or eclampsia*—**Adult:** 4 g IV in 250 ml D_5W and 4-5 g deep IM each buttock; then 4 g deep IM alternate buttock q 4 hr prn. Or, 4 g IV initially; then 1-2 g/hr IV infusion. Max, 40 g/d.

---

§ Adjust in immunocompromised patients   ¶ Adjust in debilitated patients

➤ *Hypomagnesemia, seizures*—**Adult:** 1-2 g (as 10% solution) IV over 15 min; then 1 g IM q 4-6 hr prn, per response and drug level.

➤ *Seizures, hypomagnesemia with acute nephritis in child*—**Child:** 0.2 ml/kg 50% solution IM q 4-6 hr prn, or 100-200 mg/kg 1-3% solution IV slowly.

➤ *PAT*—**Adult:** 3-4 g IV over 30 sec.

➤ *Ventricular arrhythmias*—**Adult:** 1-6 g IV over several min, then 3-20 mg/min IV × 5-48 hr.

mannitol
Osmitrol

Osmotic diuretic; diuretic
PRC: B

Available forms
Injection: 5, 10, 15, 20, 25%

Indications & dosages
➤ *Test dose for oliguria or inadequate renal function*—**Adult, child > 12 yr:** 200 mg/kg or 12.5 g as 15% or 20% IV solution over 3-5 min. Response is adequate if 30-50 ml/hr urine is produced in 2-3 hr; if inadequate, give 2nd test dose. Stop if there is no response.

➤ *Oliguria*—**Adult, child > 12 yr:** 100 g IV usually as 15% or 20% solution over 1½ to several hr.

meclizine hydrochloride
Antivert, Bonamine*, Bonine, Dramamine Less Drowsy Formula, Meni-D, Vergon

Piperazine-derivative antihistamine; antiemetic, antivertigo drug
PRC: B

Available forms
Capsules: 25, 30 mg; *Tablets:* 12.5, 25, 50 mg; *Tablets (chewable):* 25 mg

Indications & dosages
➤ *Vertigo*—**Adult:** 25-100 mg PO daily in divided doses.

➤ *Motion sickness*—**Adult:** 25-50 mg PO 1 hr before travel, then daily during trip.

medroxyprogesterone acetate
Amen, Curretab, Cycrin, Depo-Provera, Provera

Progestin; antineoplastic, hormonal contraceptive
PRC: X

Available forms
Injection (suspension): 150, 400 mg/ml; *Tablets:* 2.5, 5, 10 mg

Indications & dosages
➤ *Abnormal uterine bleeding*—**Adult:** 5-10 mg PO daily × 5-10 d starting on d 16 of menstrual cycle. If patient takes estrogen, 10 mg PO daily × 10 d starting on d 16 of cycle.

➤ *Secondary amenorrhea*—**Adult:** 5-10 mg PO daily × 5-10 d.

➤ *Endometrial or renal CA*—**Adult:** 400-1,000 mg IM wkly.

➤ *Contraception*—**Adult:** 150 mg IM q 3 mo; give 1st injection during 1st 5 d of menstrual cycle.

medroxyprogesterone acetate and estradiol cypionate
Lunelle

Estrogen and progestin; combined hormonal contraceptive
PRC: X

Available forms
Injection: 25 mg medroxyprogesterone acetate and 5 mg estradiol cypionate per 0.5 ml

Indications & dosages
➤ *Contraception*—**Women > 16 yr who have had menarche:** 0.5 ml IM. Give 1st dose within 1st 5 d of onset of normal menstrual period, within 5 d of a complete 1st trimester abortion, or ≥ 4 wk post-partum if not breast-feeding (if breast-feeding, ≥ 6 wk postpartum). Give 2nd and subsequent doses q mo (28-30 d, ≤ 33 d) after previous dose.

megestrol acetate
Megace

Progestin; antineoplastic
PRC: D

Available forms
Oral suspension: 40 mg/ml; *Tablets:* 20, 40 mg

Indications & dosages
➤ *Breast CA*—**Adult:** 40 mg PO qid.

➤ *Endometrial CA*—**Adult:** 40-320 mg PO daily in divided doses.

➤ *Significant wt loss*—**Adult:** 800 mg PO oral suspension daily.

meloxicam
Mobic

Enolic acid NSAID; anti-inflammatory, analgesic
PRC: C

Available forms
Tablets: 7.5 mg

Indications & dosages
➤ *OA*—**Adult:** 7.5 mg PO daily. Increase prn. Max, 15 mg/d.

memantine hydrochloride
Namenda

N-methyl-D-aspartate (NMDA) receptor antagonist; anti-dementia drug
PRC: B

Available forms
Tablets: 5, 10 mg

Indications & dosages
➤ *Moderate to severe Alzheimer's-type dementia*—**Adult:** Initially, 5 mg PO once

---

§ Adjust in immunocompromised patients ¶ Adjust in debilitated patients

daily. Increase by 5 mg/d q wk until target dose is reached. Max, 10 mg PO bid. Give all doses > 5 mg bid.†

meperidine hydrochloride (pethidine hydrochloride)
Demerol

Opioid; analgesic, adjunct to anesthesia
PRC: C; CSS II

Available forms

Injection: 25, 50, 75, 100 mg/ml; *Syrup:* 50 mg/5 ml; *Tablets:* 50, 100 mg

Indications & dosages

➤ *Pain*—**Adult:** 50-150 mg PO, IM, IV, or SC q 3-4 hr. **Child:** 1.1-1.8 mg/kg PO, IM, IV, or SC q 3-4 hr, or 175 mg/m² daily in 6 divided doses. Max single dose, ≤ 100 mg.†, ‡, ¶
➤ *Preop anesthesia*—**Adult:** 50-100 mg IM, IV, or SC 30-90 min preop. **Child:** 1-2.2 mg/kg IM, IV, or SC up to adult dose 30-90 min preop.

metformin hydrochloride
Glucophage, Glucophage XR, Riomet

Biguanide; antidiabetic
PRC: B

Available forms

Oral solution: 500 mg/5 ml; *Tablets:* 500, 850, 1,000 mg; *Tablets (extended-release):* 500, 750 mg

Indications & dosages

➤ *Type 2 DM*—**Adult:** 500 mg PO bid with am, pm meals; or 850 mg PO daily with am meal. With 500 mg, increase dose 500 mg/wk to max 2,500 mg (tablets) or 2,550 mg (oral solution) PO daily in divided doses prn. Or, 500 mg PO bid titrated to 850 mg bid after 2 wk. With 850 mg, increase dose 850 mg q other wk to max 2,550 mg daily in divided doses prn. Use lower dose in elderly. For extended-release, start with 500 mg PO daily with pm meal. May increase in wkly increments of 500 mg; max 2,000 mg/d.¶ **Child 10-16 yr:** 500 mg regular-release PO bid; increase in 500-mg increments wkly to max 2,000 mg/d in divided doses.¶

methadone hydrochloride
Dolophine, Methadose

Opioid; analgesic, opioid detoxification adjunct
PRC: C; CSS: II

Available forms

Injection: 10 mg/ml; *Dispersible tablets (maintenance therapy):* 40 mg; *Oral solution:* 5, 10 mg/5 ml, 10 mg/1 ml (concentrate); *Tablets:* 5, 10 mg

Indications & dosages

➤ *Pain*—**Adult:** 2.5-10 mg PO, IM, or SC q 3-4 hr prn.
➤ *Opioid withdrawal syndrome*—**Adult:** 15-40 mg PO daily. Maintenance, 20-

---

120 mg PO daily. Doses > 120 mg/d need state, federal approval.

methotrexate (amethopterin, MTX)

methotrexate sodium
Folex PFS, Mexate-AQ, Rheumatrex

Antimetabolite (cell cycle–phase specific, S phase); antineoplastic, immunosuppressant
PRC: X

Available forms
Injection: 20 mg, 50 mg, 1 g vials, lyophilized powder, preservative free; 25-mg/ml vials, preservative-free solution; 2.5-, 25-mg/ml vials, lyophilized powder, preserved; *Tablets (scored):* 2.5 mg

Indications & dosages
➤ *Trophoblastic tumors*—**Adult:** 15-30 mg PO or IM daily × 5 d. Repeat after ≥ 1 wk, based on response or toxicity.†
➤ *ALL*—**Adult, child:** 3.3 mg/m²/d PO, IM, or IV daily × 4-6 wk or until remission; then 20-30 mg/m² PO or IM wkly in 2 divided doses or 2.5 mg/kg IV q 14 d.†
➤ *Meningeal leukemia*—**Adult, child:** ≤ 12 mg/m² (max, 15 mg) intrathecally q 2-5 d until CSF is normal; then 1 more dose.†
➤ *RA*—**Adult:** Initially, 7.5 mg/wk PO as single dose or divided into 2.5 mg PO q 12 hr × 3 doses wkly. Increase gradually to optimum response. Max, 20 mg/wk. Reduce to lowest effective dose.†

methyldopa
Aldomet, Apo-Methyldopa*, Dopamet*, Novo-Medopa*

methyldopate hydrochloride
Aldomet

Centrally acting antiadrenergic; antihypertensive
PRC: B (PO), C (IV)

Available forms
methyldopa *Tablets:* 250, 500 mg; **hydrochloride** *Injection:* 250 mg/5 ml

Indications & dosages
➤ *HTN, HTN crisis*—**Adult:** 250 mg PO bid or tid in 1st 48 hr. Increase prn q 2 d. Maintenance, 500 mg-3 g daily in 2-4 divided doses; max, 3 g/d. Or, 250-500 mg diluted in D₅W IV over 30-60 min q 6 hr; max dose 1 g q 6 hr. **Child:** 10 mg/kg PO daily in 2-4 divided doses; or 20-40 mg/kg IV daily in 4 divided doses. Increase dose daily prn. Max, 65 mg/kg or 3 g daily.

---

§ Adjust in immunocompromised patients   ¶ Adjust in debilitated patients

methylphenidate hydrochloride
Concerta, Metadate CD, Metadate ER, Methylin, Methylin ER, PMS-Methylphenidate*, Ritalin, Ritalin LA, Ritalin-SR

Piperidine CNS stimulant; CNS stimulant (analeptic)
PRC: NR (C, Concerta, Metadate CD, Ritalin LA); CSS: II

Available forms
Capsules: 20 mg; *Capsules (extended-release):* 20, 30, 40 mg; *Oral solution:* 5, 10 mg/5 ml; *Tablets:* 5, 10, 20 mg; *Tablets (extended-release):* 10, 18, 20, 27, 36, 54 mg; *Tablets (sustained-release):* 20 mg

Indications & dosages
Ritalin-SR, Metadate ER, and Methylin ER tablets may be used in place of methylphenidate tablets by calculating the dose of methylphenidate in intervals of 8 hr.
➤ *ADHD (Metadate ER, Methylin, Methylin ER, Ritalin, Ritalin-SR)*—**Child ≥ 6 yr:** 5-10 mg PO daily before breakfast and lunch; increase in 5- to 10-mg increments wkly prn; max 2 mg/kg or 60 mg/d.
➤ *ADHD (Metadate CD)*—**Child ≥ 6 yr:** 20 mg PO daily before breakfast; increase in 20-mg increments wkly to max of 60 mg/d.
➤ *ADHD (Ritalin LA)*—**Child ≥ 6 yr:** 20 mg PO daily. Adjust dosage in wkly 10-mg increments to max of 60 mg daily. If previous daily dose is 10 mg bid or 20 mg sustained-release, give 20 mg PO daily. If previous daily dose is 15 mg bid,

give 30 mg PO daily. If previous daily dose is 20 mg bid or 40 mg sustained-release, give 40 mg PO daily. If previous daily dose is 30 mg bid or 60 mg sustained-release, give 60 mg PO daily.
➤ *ADHD (Concerta)*—**Child ≥ 6 yr not taking drug or taking stimulants:** Initially, 18 mg PO daily in am. Adjust wkly by 18-mg increments to max of 54 mg PO daily in am. **Child ≥ 6 yr taking this drug:** If previous daily dose is 10-15 mg or 20 mg sustained-release, give 18 mg PO q am. If previous daily dose is 20-30 mg or 40 mg sustained-release, give 36 mg PO q am. If previous daily dose 30-45 mg or 60 mg sustained-release, give 54 mg PO q am. Adjust in 18-mg increments q wk prn. Max 54 mg/d.
➤ *Narcolepsy*—**Adult:** 10 mg (Metadate ER, Methylin, Methylin ER, Ritalin, Ritalin-SR) PO bid or tid 30-45 min ac. Some patients may require 40-60 mg/d.

methylprednisolone
Medrol

methylprednisolone acetate
depMedalone 40, depMedalone 80, Depo-Medrol, Depopred-40, Depopred-80

methylprednisolone sodium succinate
A-MethaPred, Solu-Medrol

Glucocorticoid; anti-inflammatory, immunosuppressant
PRC: C

Available forms
methylprednisolone *Tablets:* 2, 4, 8, 16, 24, 32 mg; **acetate** *Injection (suspension):* 20, 40, 80 mg/ml; **sodium succinate** *Injection:* 40-, 125-, 500-, 1,000-, 2,000-mg vials

Indications & dosages
➤ *MS*—**Adult:** 200 mg PO daily × 1 wk; then 80 mg q other d × 1 mo.
➤ *Inflammation, immunosuppression*—**Adult:** 2-60 mg PO daily in 4 divided doses; or 10-80 mg acetate IM daily, or 10-250 mg succinate IM or IV up to q 4 hr. Or, 4-40 mg acetate into small joints or 20-80 mg acetate into large joints. **Child:** 0.03-0.2 mg/kg succinate or 1-6.25 mg/m² IM daily or bid.
➤ *Shock*—**Adult:** 100-250 mg succinate IV at 2-6 hr intervals; or 30 mg/kg IV, repeated q 4-6 hr prn. Continue treatment × 2-3 d or until patient is stable.

metoclopramide hydrochloride
Apo-Metoclop*, Clopra, Maxolon, Metoclopramide Intensol, Octamide, Reclomide, Reglan

Para-aminobenzoic acid derivative; antiemetic, GI stimulant
PRC: B

Available forms
Injection: 5 mg/ml; *Oral solution:* 5 mg/ 5 ml, 10 mg/ml (concentrate); *Tablets:* 5, 10 mg

Indications & dosages
➤ *Nausea, vomiting with chemo*—**Adult:** 1-2 mg/kg IV 30 min before chemo; repeat q 2 hr × 2 doses, then q 3 hr × 3 doses.
➤ *Postop nausea, vomiting*—**Adult:** 10-20 mg IM near end of procedure; then q 4-6 hr prn.
➤ *Small bowel intubation, aid in radiologic exams*—**Adult, child > 14 yr:** 10 mg IV × 1 dose over 1-2 min. **Child 6-14 yr:** 2.5-5 mg IV. **Child < 6 yr:** 0.1 mg/kg IV.
➤ *GERD*—**Adult:** 10-15 mg PO qid prn, 30 min ac and hs.

metolazone
Mykrox, Zaroxolyn

Quinazoline derivative (thiazide-like) diuretic; diuretic, antihypertensive
PRC: B

Available forms
Tablets (extended-release): 2.5, 5, 10 mg (Zaroxolyn); *Tablets (prompt-release):* 0.5 mg (Mykrox)

Indications & dosages
➤ *Edema*—**Adult:** 5-20 mg extended-release PO daily.
➤ *HTN*—**Adult:** 2.5-5 mg extended-release PO daily. Maintenance based on BP. Or, 0.5 mg prompt-release PO daily in am; increase to 1 mg PO daily.

metoprolol succinate
Toprol-XL

metoprolol tartrate
Apo-Metoprolol*, Lopressor

Beta blocker; antihypertensive, adjunctive treatment for acute MI
PRC: C

Available forms
succinate *Tablets (extended-release):* 25, 50, 100, 200 mg; **tartrate** *Injection:* 1 mg/ml in 5-ml ampule; *Tablets:* 50, 100 mg

Indications & dosages
➤ *HTN*—**Adult:** 100 mg PO in 1 dose or divided doses; maintenance, 100-450 mg/d in 2-3 divided doses. Or, 50-100 mg extended-release tablet daily; max, 400 mg/d.
➤ *Acute MI*—**Adult:** 5-mg tartrate IV bolus q 2 min × 3 doses. Then, 15 min after last dose, 25-50 mg PO q 6 hr × 48 hr. Maintenance, 100 mg PO bid.
➤ *Angina*—**Adult:** 100 mg PO daily in 2 divided doses or 100 mg extended-release tablet daily. Maintenance, 100-400 mg/d.
➤ *Stable, symptomatic HF from ischemia, HTN, or cardiomyopathy*—**Adult:** 25 mg extended-release tablet PO daily × 2 wk. Double dose q 2 wk as tolerated to max of 200 mg daily. In patient with more severe HF, start with 12.5 mg PO daily × 2 wk.

metronidazole (systemic)
Apo-Metronidazole*, Flagyl, Protostat, Trikacide*

metronidazole hydrochloride
Flagyl IV RTU, Metro IV, Novonidazol*

Nitroimidazole; antibacterial, anti-protozoal, amebicide
PRC: B

Available forms
Capsules: 375 mg; *Injection:* 5 mg/ml; *Powder for injection:* 500-mg single-dose vial; *Tablets:* 250, 500 mg; *Tablets (extended-release):* 750 mg

Indications & dosages
➤ *Intestinal amebiasis*—**Adult:** 750 mg PO tid × 5-10 d. **Child:** 30-50 mg/kg/d (in 3 doses) × 10 d.
➤ *Trichomoniasis*—**Adult:** 250 mg PO tid × 7 d or 2 g PO in 1 dose; repeat after 4-6 wk. **Child:** 5 mg/kg dose PO tid × 7 d.
➤ *Refractory trichomoniasis*—**Adult:** 250 or 500 mg PO bid × 10 or 7 d, respectively.
➤ *Bacterial infection from anaerobic microorganisms*—**Adult:** Loading, 15 mg/kg IV over 1 hr. Maintenance, 7.5 mg/kg IV or PO q 6 hr. First maintenance dose 6 hr after loading dose. Max, 4 g/d.
➤ *Contaminated colorectal surgery*—**Adult:** 15 mg/kg IV over 30-60 min 1 hr preop; then 7.5 mg/kg IV over 30-60 min at 6 and 12 hr after 1st dose.

---

mexiletine hydrochloride
Mexitil

Lidocaine analogue, sodium channel antagonist; ventricular antiarrhythmic
PRC: C

Available forms
Capsules: 100*, 150, 200, 250 mg

Indications & dosages
➤ *Ventricular arrhythmias*—**Adult:** 200 mg PO q 8 hr. May increase to 50-100 mg q 8 hr. Or, loading dose 400 mg with maintenance dose 200 mg q 8 hr. Max, 1,200 mg/d.

miconazole nitrate
Micatin, Monistat 3, Monistat 7, Monistat-Derm

Imidazole derivative; antifungal
PRC: C

Available forms
Cream, ointment, powder, solution, spray, vaginal cream: 2%; *Vaginal suppository:* 100, 200 mg

Indications & dosages
➤ *Tinea pedis, cruris, corporis*—**Adult, child:** Apply or spray sparingly bid × 2-4 wk.
➤ *Vulvovaginal candidiasis*—**Adult:** 1 applicator or 100-mg suppository (Monistat 7) inserted intravaginally hs × 7 d; repeat course prn. Or, 200-mg suppository (Monistat 3) intravaginally hs × 3 d.

midazolam hydrochloride
Versed

Benzodiazepine; preop sedative, conscious sedation, adjunctive treatment for induction of general anesthesia, amnestic
PRC: D; CSS: IV

Available forms
Injection: 1, 5 mg/ml

Indications & dosages
➤ *Preop sedation*—**Adult:** 0.07-0.08 mg/kg IM 1 hr preop. ¶
➤ *Conscious sedation*—**Adult:** 1-2 mg slow IV injection before procedure. ¶
➤ *Induction of general anesthesia*—**Adult:** 0.15-0.35 mg/kg over 20-30 sec. Then, increments of 25% initial dose prn. Max, 0.6 mg/kg. **Unpremedicated adult ≥ 55 yr:** Initially, 0.3 mg/kg. ¶

mifepristone
Mifeprex

Synthetic steroid; anti-progestin, abortifacient
PRC: NR

Available forms
Tablets: 200 mg

Indications & dosages
➤ *Termination of intrauterine pregnancy through 49th d*—**Adult:** 600 mg PO as 1 dose. On d 3, unless abortion is con-

---

firmed by exam or ultrasound, 400 mcg misoprostol PO × 1 dose.

miglitol
Glyset

Alpha-glucosidase inhibitor; antidiabetic
PRC: B

Available forms
Tablets: 25, 50, 100 mg

Indications & dosages
➤ *Type 2 DM*—**Adult:** 25 mg PO tid at start of each main meal; increase prn after 4-8 wk to 50 mg PO tid. May be further increased after 3 mo based on HbA$_{1c}$; max, 100 mg PO tid.

milrinone lactate
Primacor

Bipyridine phosphodiesterase inhibitor; inotropic vasodilator
PRC: C

Available forms
Injection: 1 mg/ml; *Injection (premixed):* 200 mcg/ml in D$_5$W

Indications & dosages
➤ *HF*—**Adult:** Loading dose 50 mcg/kg IV slowly over 10 min; then continue infusion of 0.375-0.75 mcg/kg/min.†

minocycline hydrochloride
Alti-Minocycline*, Apo-Minocycline*, Dynacin, Minocin, Novo-Minocycline*, PMS-Minocycline

Tetracycline; antibiotic
PRC: D

Available forms
Capsules: 50, 75, 100 mg; *Capsules (pellet-filled):* 50, 100 mg; *Injection:* 100 mg/vial; *Tablets:* 50, 75, 100 mg

Indications & dosages
➤ *Infection*—**Adult:** 200 mg IV; then 100 mg IV q 12 hr. Max, 400 mg/d. Or, 200 mg PO; then 100 mg PO q 12 hr. Or, 100-200 mg PO; then 50 mg qid.† **Child > 8 yr:** 4 mg/kg PO or IV; then 2 mg/kg q 12 hr IV in 500- to 1,000-ml solution without calcium over 6 hr.†
➤ *Gonorrhea in PCN-allergic patient*—**Adult:** 200 mg PO; then 100 mg q 12 hr ≥ 4 d.†
➤ *Syphilis in PCN-allergic patient*—**Adult:** 200 mg PO; then 100 mg q 12 hr × 10-15 d.†
➤ *Meningococcal carrier state*—**Adult:** 100 mg PO q 12 hr × 5 d.†
➤ *Uncomplicated urethral, endocervical, rectal infection from* Chlamydia trachomatis—100 mg PO q 12 hr × ≥ 7 d.†

minoxidil
Loniten

Peripheral vasodilator; antihypertensive
PRC: C

---

*Canadian   †Adjust in renal impairment   ‡Adjust in liver impairment

Available forms
Tablets: 2.5, 10 mg

Indications & dosages
➤ *HTN*—**Adult, child ≥ 12 yr:** 5 mg PO daily. Effective dose, 10-40 mg/d. Max, 100 mg/d. **Child < 12 yr:** 0.2 mg/kg PO daily; max, 5 mg/d. Effective dose, 0.25-1 mg/kg/d. Max, 50 mg/d.

mirtazapine
Remeron, Remeron SolTab

Piperazinoazepine; tetracyclic antidepressant
PRC: C

Available forms
Tablets: 15, 30, 45 mg; *Tablets (orally disintegrating):* 15, 30, 45 mg

Indications & dosages
Depression—**Adult:** 15 mg PO hs. Maintenance, 15-45 mg/d. Adjust dose at ≥ 1-2 wk.

misoprostol
Cytotec

Prostaglandin E$_1$ analogue; antiulcerative, gastric mucosal protectant
PRC: X

Available forms
Tablets: 100, 200 mcg

Indications & dosages
➤ *Prevention of NSAID-induced gastric ulcers*—**Adult:** 200 mcg PO qid (last dose hs) with food; if not tolerated, decrease to 100 mcg qid.

moexipril hydrochloride
Univasc

ACE inhibitor; antihypertensive
PRC: C (D, 2nd and 3rd trimesters)

Available forms
Tablets: 7.5, 15 mg

Indications & dosages
➤ *HTN*—**Adult:** 7.5 mg (3.75 mg if patient is on diuretic) PO daily 1 hr ac. Maintenance, 7.5-30 mg daily, in 1 or 2 divided doses 1 hr ac.†

montelukast sodium
Singulair

Leukotriene receptor antagonist; antiasthmatic
PRC: B

Available forms
Granules: 4-mg packet; *Tablets (chewable):* 4, 5 mg; *Tablets (film-coated):* 10 mg

Indications & dosages
➤ *Asthma, seasonal allergic rhinitis*—**Adult, child ≥ 15 yr:** 10 mg film-coated PO daily q pm. **Child 6-14 yr:** 5 mg (chewable) PO daily q pm. **Child 2-5 yr:** 4 mg chewable or 1 packet granules PO daily q pm.
➤ *Asthma*—**Child 12-23 mo:** 1 packet of 4-mg granules PO daily q pm.

---

§ Adjust in immunocompromised patients   ¶ Adjust in debilitated patients

morphine hydrochloride
Morphitec*, M.O.S.*

morphine sulfate
Astramorph PF, Avinza, Duramorph, Epimorph*, Infumorph 200, Morphine H.P.*, MS Contin, Roxanol

Opioid; opioid analgesic
PRC: C; CSS: II

Available forms
hydrochloride *Oral solution*, syrup*:* 1, 5, 10, 20, 50 mg/ml; *Suppository*:* 10, 20, 30 mg; *Tablets*:* 10, 20, 40, 60 mg; *Tablets (extended-release)*:* 30, 60 mg; **sulfate** *Capsules (extended-release):* 30, 60, 90, 120 mg; *Injection (with preservative):* 0.5, 1, 2, 4, 5, 8, 10, 15, 25, 50 mg/ml; *Injection (without preservative):* 0.5, 1, 10, 15, 25 mg/ml; *Oral solution:* 10, 20, 100 mg/5 ml, 20 mg/ml (concentrate); *Solution tablets:* 10, 15, 30 mg; *Suppository:* 5, 10, 20, 30 mg; *Tablets:* 15, 30 mg; *Tablets (extended-release):* 15, 30, 60, 100, 200 mg

Indications & dosages
➤ *Pain—***Adult:** 5-20 mg SC or IM; or 2.5-15 mg IV q 4 hr prn; or 10-30 mg PO or 10-20 mg PR q 4 hr prn. For continuous IV, loading dose 15 mg IV; then infuse 0.8-10 mg/hr. Or, 15-30 mg extended-release tablet PO q 8-12 hr or 30 mg extended-release capsule PO daily. Epidural injection, 5 mg; then, if no adequate pain relief is achieved within 1 hr, additional doses of 1-2 mg. Max total epidural dose, ≤ 10 mg/24 hr. **Child:** 0.1-

0.2 mg/kg SC or IM q 4 hr. Max single dose, 15 mg.

moxifloxacin hydrochloride (ophthalmic)
Vigamox

Fluoroquinolone; antibiotic
PRC: C

Available forms
Solution: 0.5%

Indications & dosages
➤ *Bacterial conjunctivitis—***Adult, child ≥ 1 yr:** 1 drop into affected eye tid × 7 d.

moxifloxacin hydrochloride (systemic)
Avelox, Avelox IV

Fluoroquinolone; antibiotic
PRC: C

Available forms
Infusion: 400 mg/250 ml; *Tablets (film-coated):* 400 mg

Indications & dosages
➤ *Sinusitis—***Adult:** 400 mg PO or IV daily × 10 d.
➤ *Chronic bronchitis exacerbation—***Adult:** 400 mg PO or IV daily × 5 d.
➤ *Community-acquired pneumonia—***Adult:** 400 mg PO or IV daily × 7-14 d.
➤ *Uncomplicated skin and skin-structure infection—***Adult:** 400 mg PO or IV daily × 7 d.

nadolol
Corgard

Beta blocker; antihypertensive, anti-anginal
PRC: C

Available forms
Tablets: 20, 40, 80, 120, 160 mg

Indications & dosages
➤ *Angina*—**Adult:** 40 mg PO daily. Increase by 40-80 mg prn. Maintenance, 40-80 mg/d. †
➤ *HTN*—**Adult:** 40 mg PO daily. Increase by 40-80 mg prn. Maintenance, 40-80 mg/d. Up to 320 mg may be needed. †

nafcillin sodium

Penicillinase-resistant PCN; antibiotic
PRC: B

Available forms
Injection for IV infusion: 1, 2 g

Indications & dosages
➤ *Systemic infections caused by susceptible organisms (methicillin-sensitive* Staphylococcus aureus*)*—**Adult:** 500 mg-1 g IV q 4 hr depending on the severity of the infection. **Infant, child > 1 mo:** 50-200 mg/kg/d IV in divided doses q 4-6 hr depending on the severity of the infection. **Neonate > 7 d, ≤ 2 kg:** 25 mg/kg IV q 8 hr. **Neonate > 7 d, > 2 kg:** 25 mg/kg IV q 6 hr. **Neonate ≤ 7 d, ≤ 2 kg:** 25 mg/kg

IV q 12 hr. **Neonate ≤ 7 d, >2 kg:** 25 mg/kg IV q 8 hr.
➤ *Meningitis*—**Adult:** 100-200 mg/kg/d IV in divided doses q 4-6 hr. **Neonate > 7 d, ≤ 2 kg:** 50 mg/kg IV q 8 hr. **Neonate > 7 d, > 2 kg:** 50 mg/kg IV q 6 hr. **Neonate ≤ 7 d, ≤ 2 kg:** 50 mg/kg IV q 12 hr. **Neonate ≤ 7 d, > 2 kg:** 50 mg/kg IV q 8 hr.
➤ *Osteomyelitis*—**Adult:** 1-2 g IV q 4 hr × 4-8 wk. **Infant, child > 1 mo:** 100-200 mg/kg/d in divided doses q 4-6 hr.
➤ *Native valve endocarditis*—**Adult:** 2 g IV q 4 hr × 4-6 wk with gentamicin. **Infant, child > 1 mo:** 100-200 mg/kg/d in divided doses q 4-6 hr.

nalbuphine hydrochloride
Nubain

Opioid agonist-antagonist, opioid partial agonist; analgesic, adjunct to anesthesia
PRC: NR

Available forms
Injection: 10, 20 mg/ml

Indications & dosages
➤ *Pain*—**Adult:** Average-weight (70-kg) patient, 10-20 mg SC, IM, or IV q 3-6 hr prn. Max, 160 mg/d.
➤ *Adjunct to anesthesia*—**Adult:** 0.3-3 mg/kg IV over 10-15 min; then maintenance dose, 0.25-0.5 mg/kg IV prn.

naloxone hydrochloride
Narcan

Opioid antagonist; opioid antagonist
PRC: B

Available forms
Injection: 0.02, 0.4, 1 mg/ml

Indications & dosages
➤ *Opioid-induced respiratory depression*—**Adult:** 0.4-2 mg IV, SC, or IM. Repeat q 2-3 min prn. Reconsider diagnosis if no response after 10 min. **Child:** 0.01 mg/kg IV; then 2nd dose of 0.1 mg/kg IV prn. If no IV, give IM or SC in divided doses. **Neonate:** 0.01 mg/kg IV, IM, or SC. Repeat dose q 2-3 min prn.
➤ *Postop opioid depression*—**Adult:** 0.1-0.2 mg IV q 2-3 min until desired degree of reversal is reached. Repeat dose within 1-2 hr if needed. **Child:** 0.005-0.01 mg IV. Repeat q 2-3 min until desired degree of reversal is reached.
➤ *Opiate-induced asphyxia neonatorum*—**Neonate:** 0.01 mg/kg IV via umbilical vein. Repeat q 2-3 min until desired degree of reversal is reached.

naltrexone hydrochloride
Depade, ReVia

Opioid antagonist; opioid detoxification adjunct
PRC: C

Available forms
Tablets: 50 mg

Indications & dosages
➤ *Maintenance of opioid-free state in detoxified patient*—**Adult:** 25 mg PO. If no withdrawal signs after 1 hr, give additional 25 mg. When patient is using 50 mg q 24 hr, use flexible maintenance schedule.
➤ *Alcohol dependence*—**Adult:** 50 mg PO daily.

naproxen
EC-Naprosyn, Naprosyn, Naprosyn SR*, Novo-Naprox*

naproxen sodium
Aleve, Anaprox, Anaprox DS, Apo-Napro-Na*, Naprelan, Synflex*

NSAID; nonopioid analgesic, antipyretic, anti-inflammatory
PRC: B

Available forms
naproxen *Oral suspension:* 125 mg/5 ml; *Tablets:* 250, 375, 500 mg; *Tablets (delayed-release):* 250, 375, 500 mg; *Tablets (extended-release):* 750, 1,000 mg; **sodium** *Tablets:* 220 mg (equivalent to 200 mg naproxen); *Tablets (film-coated):* 275 (equivalent to 250 mg naproxen), 550 (equivalent to 500 mg naproxen) mg; *Tablets (extended-release):* 412.5 (equivalent to 375 mg naproxen), 550 mg (equivalent to 500 mg naproxen).

Indications & dosages
➤ *RA, OA, ankylosing spondylitis, pain, dysmenorrhea, tendinitis, bursitis*—**Adult:** 250-500 mg naproxen bid; max, 1.5 g/d. Or, 375-500 mg delayed-release (EC-Naprosyn) bid; or 750-1,000 mg

extended-release (Naprelan) bid; or 275-550 mg sodium bid.
➤ *Juvenile arthritis*—**Child:** 10 mg/kg PO in 2 divided doses.
➤ *Gout*—**Adult:** 750 mg naproxen PO, then 250 mg q 8 hr until attack subsides. Or, 825 mg sodium, then 275 mg q 8 hr until attack subsides; or 1,000-1,500 mg/d extended-release (Naprelan) on 1st d, then 1,000 mg/d.
➤ *Pain, dysmenorrhea*—**Adult:** 500 mg naproxen PO, then 250 mg q 6-8 hr, max 1.25 g/d. Or, 550 mg sodium, then 275 mg q 6-8 hr, max 1.375 g/d; or 1,000 mg extended-release (Naprelan) daily.

nateglinide
Starlix

Amino acid derivative; antidiabetic
PRC: C

Available forms
Tablets: 60, 120 mg

Indications & dosages
➤ *Type 2 DM, alone or with metformin or a thiazolidinedione*—**Adult:** 120 mg PO tid, ≤ 30 min ac. If HbA$_{1c}$ is near goal when treatment starts, 60 mg PO tid.

nefazodone hydrochloride
Serzone

Phenylpiperazine; antidepressant
PRC: C

Available forms
Tablets: 50, 100, 150, 200, 250 mg

Indications & dosages
➤ *Depression*—**Adult:** 200 mg/d PO in 2 divided doses.¶ Increase 100-200 mg/d at ≥ 1 wk prn. Range, 300-600 mg/d. **Elderly:** 50 mg PO bid.

nelfinavir mesylate
Viracept

HIV protease inhibitor; antiviral
PRC: B

Available forms
Powder for suspension: 50 mg/g powder in 144-g bottle; *Tablets:* 250, 625 mg

Indications & dosages
➤ *HIV infection*—**Adult:** 750 mg PO tid. Or, 1,250 mg PO bid with meal. **Child 2-13 yr:** 20-30 mg/kg PO tid. Max 750 mg tid.

neostigmine bromide
Prostigmin

neostigmine methylsulfate
Prostigmin

Cholinesterase inhibitor; muscle stimulant
PRC: C

Available forms
bromide *Tablets:* 15 mg; **methylsulfate** *Injection:* 0.25, 0.5, 1 mg/ml

Indications & dosages
➤ *Myasthenia gravis*—**Adult:** 0.5 mg SC or IM. Or, 15-375 mg/d PO. **Child:** 7.5-15 mg PO tid or qid.

§ Adjust in immunocompromised patients ¶ Adjust in debilitated patients

➤ *Diagnosis of myasthenia gravis*—
Adult: 0.022 mg/kg IM 30 min after atropine IM. **Child:** 0.025-0.04 mg/kg IM after atropine SC.
➤ *Postop abdominal distention and bladder atony*—**Adult:** 0.5-1 mg IM or SC q 3 hr × 5 doses after bladder is emptied.
➤ *Antidote for nondepolarizing neuromuscular blockers*—**Adult:** 0.5-2 mg IV slowly. Repeat prn. Max 5 mg. Before antidote dose, give atropine IV.

nesiritide
Natrecor

Human B-type natriuretic peptide;
inotropic vasodilator
PRC: C

Available forms
Injection: 1.5 mg sterile, lyophilized powder single-dose vials

Indications & dosages
➤ *Acutely decompensated and symptomatic HF*—**Adult:** 2 mcg/kg IV over 60 sec; then continuous infusion of 0.01 mcg/kg/min.

nevirapine
Viramune

Nonnucleoside reverse transcriptase
inhibitor; antiviral
PRC: C

Available forms
PO suspension: 50 mg/5 ml; *Tablets:* 200 mg

Indications & dosages
➤ *HIV-1 infection*—**Adult:** 200 mg PO daily × 1st 14 d, then 200 mg PO bid.
Child ≥ 8 yr: 4 mg/kg PO daily × 14 d, then 4 mg/kg PO bid. Max 400 mg/d.
Child 2 mo-8 yr: 4 mg/kg PO daily × 14 d, then 7 mg/kg PO bid. Max, 400 mg/d.

niacin (nicotinic acid, vitamin B_3)
Niacor, Nico-400, Nicobid, Nicolar

niacinamide (nicotinamide)

B-complex vitamin; vitamin B_3, antilipemic, peripheral vasodilator
PRC: C

Available forms
niacin *Capsules (extended-release):* 125, 250, 400, 500 mg; *Elixir:* 50 mg/5 ml; *Tablets:* 50, 100, 250, 500 mg; *Tablets (extended-release):* 250, 500, 750 mg;
niacinamide *Tablets:* 50, 100, 500 mg

Indications & dosages
➤ *Pellagra*—**Adult:** 300-500 mg PO daily in divided doses. **Child:** 100-300 mg PO daily in divided doses.
➤ *Hyperlipidemia (niacin only)*—**Adult:** 1-2 g PO bid or tid with meals or pc; max, 6 g/d.

---

nicardipine
Cardene, Cardene I.V., Cardene SR

Calcium channel blocker; antianginal, antihypertensive
PRC: C

Available forms
Capsules (immediate-release): 20, 30 mg; *Capsules (sustained-release):* 30, 45, 60 mg; *Injection:* 2.5 mg/ml

Indications & dosages
➤ *Angina, HTN*—**Adult:** 20 mg immediate-release PO tid. Adjust to response q 3 d. Range (immediate-release), 20-40 mg tid. Range(sustained-release), 30-60 mg bid.
➤ *HTN (short-term)*—**Adult:** If unable to take PO, 5 mg/hr IV; titrate to 2.5 mg/hr q 15 min; max, 15 mg/hr.

nifedipine
Adalat, Adalat CC, Apo-Nifed*, Nifedical XL, Nu-Nifed*, Procardia, Procardia XL

Calcium channel blocker; antianginal, antihypertensive
PRC: C

Available forms
Capsules: 10, 20 mg; *Tablets (extended-release):* 30, 60, 90 mg

Indications & dosages
➤ *Prinzmetal's angina*—**Adult:** 10 mg PO tid. Range 10-20 mg tid. Max, 180 mg/d.

➤ *HTN*—**Adult:** 30 or 60 mg PO daily. Adjust over 7-14 d. Doses > 90 mg (for Adalat CC) and > 120 mg (for Procardia XL, Nifedical XL) not recommended.

nisoldipine
Sular

Calcium channel blocker; antihypertensive
PRC: C

Available forms
Tablets (extended-release): 10, 20, 30, 40 mg

Indications & dosages
➤ *HTN*—**Adult:** 20 mg PO daily ‡; increase by 10 mg/wk or at longer intervals prn. Maintenance, 20-40 mg/d. Max, 60 mg/d. **Elderly:** Initially ≤ 10 mg PO daily.

nitazoxanide
Alinia, Cryptaz

Antiprotozoan; antidiarrheal, anti-infective
PRC: B

Available forms
Powder for injection: 100 mg/5 ml in 60-ml bottle

Indications & dosages
➤ *Diarrhea caused by* Cryptosporidium parvum *and* Giardia lamblia—**Child 4-11 yr:** 10 ml (200 mg) PO q 12 hr × 3 d with food. **Child 1-4 yr:** 5 ml (100 mg) PO q 12 hr × 3 d with food.

---

§ Adjust in immunocompromised patients ¶ Adjust in debilitated patients

nitrofurantoin macrocrystals
Macrobid, Macrodantin

nitrofurantoin microcrystals
Furadantin

Nitrofuran; urinary tract anti-infective
PRC: B

Available forms
macrocrystals *Capsules:* 25, 50, 100 mg; **microcrystals** *Oral suspension:* 25 mg/ 5 ml

Indications & dosages
➤ *UTI*—**Adult, child > 12 yr:** 50-100 mg PO qid with meals and hs. Or, 100 mg Macrobid PO q 12 hr × 7 d. **Child 1 mo-12 yr:** 5-7 mg/kg PO daily divided qid.
➤ *Suppression therapy*—**Adult:** 50-100 mg PO q hs. **Child:** 1 mg/kg PO daily in 1 dose hs or divided into 2 doses.

nitroglycerin (glyceryl trinitrate)
Nitro-Bid, Nitrocine, Nitrodisc, Nitro-Dur, Nitrogard, Nitroglyn, Nitrolingual, Nitrostat, Transderm-Nitro, Tridil

Nitrate; antianginal, vasodilator
PRC: C

Available forms
Aerosol (translingual): 0.4-mg metered spray; *Capsules (sustained-release):* 2.5, 6.5, 9, 13 mg; *Injection:* 0.5, 5 mg/ml; *Tablets (buccal):* 1, 2, 3 mg; *Tablets (SL):* 0.3, 0.4, 0.6 mg; *Tablets (sustained-release):* 2.6, 6.5, 9, 13 mg; *Topical ointment:* 2%; *Transdermal:* 0.1, 0.2, 0.3, 0.4, 0.6, 0.8 mg/hr release rate

Indications & dosages
➤ *Angina prophylaxis*—**Adult:** 2.5 mg or 2.6 mg sustained-release capsule q 8-12 hr. Or, 2% ointment, ½- 5 inches. Or, transdermal disc or pad 0.2-0.4 mg/hr daily.
➤ *Acute angina, angina prophylaxis*—**Adult:** 1 tablet SL. Repeat q 5 min prn, × 15 min. Or, use Nitrolingual, 1 or 2 sprays into mouth. Repeat q 3-5 min prn, to max 3 doses in 15 min. Or, 1-3 mg transmucosally q 3-5 hr while awake.
➤ *HTN, HF, angina, control HTN during surgery, produce controlled hypotension during surgery*—**Adult:** 5 mcg/min; increase prn by 5 mcg/min q 3-5 min until response.

nitroprusside sodium
Nitropress

Vasodilator; antihypertensive
PRC: C

Available forms
Injection: 50 mg/vial in 2-, 5-ml vials

Indications & dosages
➤ *HTN emergencies*—**Adult, child:** 50-mg vial diluted with 2-3 ml D_5W and added to 250, 500, or 1,000 ml D_5W; infuse at 0.3-10 mcg/kg/min, titrate to BP. Max rate, 10 mcg/kg/min.

➤ *HF*—**Adult, child:** IV infusion titrated to cardiac output and BP. Same dose range as for HTN emergencies.

norepinephrine bitartrate
Levophed

Adrenergic; vasopressor
PRC: C

Available forms
Injection: 1 mg/ml

Indications & dosages
➤ *Acute hypotension*—**Adult:** 8-12 mcg/min IV infusion, titrate to maintain normal BP. Maintenance, 2-4 mcg/min. **Child:** 2 mcg/m²/min IV infusion. Titrate prn.

norethindrone
Camilla, Errin, Micronor, Nora-BE, Nor-QD

norethindrone acetate
Aygestin, Norlutate

Progestin; hormonal contraceptive
PRC: X

Available forms
norethindrone *Tablets:* 0.35 mg; **acetate** *Tablets:* 5 mg

Indications & dosages
➤ *Amenorrhea, abnormal uterine bleeding*—**Adult:** 2.5-20 mg PO daily on d 5-25 of menstrual cycle.
➤ *Endometriosis*—**Adult:** 5-10 mg PO daily × 14 d; then increase by 2.5-5 mg/d q 2 wk up to 15 mg/d.

➤ *Contraception*—**Adult:** 0.35 mg norethindrone PO on d 1 of menstruation; then 0.35 mg/d.

nortriptyline hydrochloride
Aventyl, Pamelor

TCA; antidepressant
PRC: D

Available forms
Capsules: 10, 25, 50, 75 mg; *Oral solution:* 10 mg/5 ml (4% alcohol)

Indications & dosages
➤ *Depression*—**Adult:** 25 mg PO tid or qid; increase to max 150 mg/d. Entire dose may be given hs. Monitor level for doses > 100 mg/d. **Elderly:** 30-50 mg PO daily in 1 dose or 2 divided doses.

nystatin
Mycostatin, Nadostine*, Nilstat, Nystex

Polyene macrolide; antifungal
PRC: C

Available forms
Cream, ointment, powder: 100,000 units/g; *Lozenges:* 200,000 units; *Oral suspension:* 100,000 units/ml; 50, 150, 500 million units; 1, 2 billion units; *Tablets:* 500,000 units; *Troche:* 200,000 units; *Vaginal tablets:* 100,000 units

Indications & dosages
➤ *Intestinal candidiasis*—**Adult:** 500,000-1 million units as PO tablet tid.

§ Adjust in immunocompromised patients   ¶ Adjust in debilitated patients

➤ *Oral infection*—**Adult, child:** 400,000-600,000 units oral suspension qid. **Infant:** 200,000 units oral suspension qid. **Neonate, premature infant:** 100,000 units oral suspension qid.
➤ *Vaginal yeast infection*—**Adult:** 100,000 units (tablet) high into vagina daily × 14 d.

ofloxacin
Floxin

Fluoroquinolone; antibiotic
PRC: C

Available forms
Tablets (film-coated): 200, 300, 400 mg

Indications & dosages
➤ *Lower respiratory tract infection*—**Adult:** 400 mg PO q 12 hr × 10 d.†
➤ *Cervicitis, urethritis*—**Adult:** 300 mg PO q 12 hr × 7 d.†
➤ *Gonorrhea*—**Adult:** 400 mg PO in 1 dose with doxycycline.†
➤ *Skin infection*—**Adult:** 400 mg PO q 12 hr × 10 d.†
➤ *Cystitis, UTI*—**Adult:** 200 mg PO q 12 hr × 3-7 d.†
➤ *Prostatitis*—**Adult:** 300 mg PO q 12 hr × 6 wk.†
➤ *PID (outpatient)*—**Adult:** 400 mg PO q 12 hr × 14 d.†

olanzapine
Zyprexa, Zyprexa Zydis

Dibenzapine derivative; antipsychotic
PRC: C

Available forms
Tablets: 2.5, 5, 7.5, 10, 15, 20 mg; *Tablets (orally disintegrating):* 5, 10, 15, 20 mg

Indications & dosages
➤ *Acute mania (bipolar I disorder)*—**Adult:** 10-15 mg PO daily. Adjust dose 5 mg/d at intervals of ≥ 24 hr prn. Max, 20 mg/d. Duration, 3-4 wk.¶
➤ *Long-term treatment of bipolar I disorder*—**Adult:** 5-20 mg PO daily.¶
➤ *Acute mania (bipolar I disorder) with lithium or valproate*—**Adult:** 10 mg PO daily. Usual range, 5-20 mg daily. Duration, 6 wk.¶
➤ *Schizophrenia*—**Adult:** 5-10 mg PO daily. Adjust dose 5 mg/d at intervals of ≥ 1 wk. Target dose, 10 mg/d. In patients prone to hypotensive reactions, in those who have risk factors for slower metabolism of drug (nonsmoking females > 65), and in those who are sensitive to drug, starting dose is 5 mg PO. Adjust dose cautiously in these patients. Max for all patients, 20 mg/d.¶

olmesartan medoxomil
Benicar

Angiotensin II receptor antagonist; antihypertensive
PRC: C (first trimester) and D (second and third trimesters)

Available forms
Tablets: 5, 20, 40 mg

Indications & dosages
➤ *HTN*—**Adult:** 20 mg PO daily in patients who aren't volume-contracted. May

---

increase dose to 40 mg PO daily if BP isn't reduced after 2 wk of therapy.†

omalizumab
Xolair

Monoclonal antibody; antiasthmatic
PRC: B

Available forms
Powder for injection: 150 mg in 5-ml vial

Indications & dosages
➤ *Allergic asthma in patients whose symptoms aren't adequately controlled by inhaled corticosteroids*—**Adult, child ≥ 12 yr:** 150-375 mg SC q 2 or 4 wk. Dosage varies with pretreatment immunoglobulin E level (IU/ml) and patient's wt. Divide doses larger than 150 mg between > 1 injection site.

omeprazole
Losec*, Prilosec, Prilosec OTC

Proton pump inhibitor; gastric acid suppressant
PRC: C

Available forms
Capsules (delayed-release): 10, 20, 40 mg; *Tablets (delayed-release):* 20 mg

Indications & dosages
➤ *Esophagitis, GERD*—**Adult:** 20 mg PO daily × 4-8 wk.‡
➤ *Frequent heartburn (≥ 2 d/wk)*—**Adult:** 20 mg (Prilosec OTC) PO once daily before breakfast × 14 d. May repeat 14-d course q 4 mo.‡

➤ *Hypersecretory conditions*—**Adult:** 60 mg PO daily; adjust to response. If dose > 80 mg, give in divided doses.‡
➤ *Duodenal ulcer*—**Adult:** 20 mg PO daily × 4-8 wk.‡
➤ *Active benign gastric ulcer*—**Adult:** 40 mg PO daily × 4-8 wk.‡
➤ Helicobacter pylori *infection*—**Adult:** 40 mg PO q am with clarithromycin × 14 d; then 20 mg daily × 14 d. Or, 20 mg bid with clarithromycin and amoxicillin × 10 d; then 20 mg of omeprazole daily × 18 d.‡

ondansetron hydrochloride
Zofran, Zofran ODT

Serotonin (5-HT$_3$) receptor antagonist; antiemetic
PRC: B

Available forms
Injection: 2 mg/ml; *Oral solution:* 4 mg/5 ml; *Premixed injection:* 32 mg/50 ml; *Tablets:* 4, 8, 24 mg; *Tablets (orally disintegrating):* 4, 8 mg

Indications & dosages
➤ *Nausea, vomiting with chemo*—**Adult, child ≥ 12 yr:** 8 mg PO 30 min before chemo. Then, 8 mg PO 8 hr after 1st dose, then 8 mg q 12 hr × 1-2 d. Or, 32 mg/15 min IV 30 min before chemo; or, 0.15 mg/kg IV over 15 min, given 30 min before chemo and repeat 4 and 8 hr after 1st dose.‡ **Child 4-12 yr:** 4 mg PO 30 min before chemo. Then 4 mg PO 4 and 8 hr later, then 4 mg q 8 hr × 1-2 d. Or, 3 doses of 0.15 mg/kg IV, as for adult.‡

---

§ Adjust in immunocompromised patients   ¶ Adjust in debilitated patients

➤ *To prevent nausea, vomiting with highly emetogenic chemo*—**Adult:** 24 mg PO 30 min before giving single-day chemo.‡
➤ *Nausea, vomiting with radiation*—**Adult:** 8 mg PO tid. ‡

oseltamivir phosphate
Tamiflu

Neuraminidase inhibitor; antiviral
PRC: C

Available forms
Capsules: 75 mg; *Oral suspension:* 12 mg/ml

Indications & dosages
➤ *Symptomatic influenza ≤ 2 d*—**Adult, child ≥ 13 yr:** 75 mg PO bid × 5 d. †
➤ *To prevent influenza after close contact with infected person*—**Adult, child ≥ 13 yr:** 75 mg PO daily within 2 d of exposure and lasting ≥ 7 d. †
➤ *To prevent influenza during community outbreak*—**Adult, child ≥ 13 yr:** 75 mg PO daily × ≤ 6 wk.†
➤ *Influenza*—**Child ≥ 1 yr: ≤ 15 kg:** 30 mg oral suspension PO bid. † **> 15-23 kg:** 45 mg oral suspension PO bid. † **> 23-40 kg:** 60 mg oral suspension PO bid. † **> 40 kg:** 75 mg oral suspension PO bid. †

oxaliplatin
Eloxatin

Alkylating drug; antineoplastic
PRC: D

Available forms
Injection: 50- or 100-mg vials

Indications & dosages
➤ *Advanced colon or rectal cancer with 5-fluorouracil (5-FU) and leucovorin*—**Adult:** On d one, 85 mg/m² oxaliplatin IV in 250-500 ml D_5W and 200 mg/m² leucovorin IV in D_5W, given at the same time over 120 min, in separate bags using a Y-line, followed by 400 mg/m² 5-FU IV bolus over 2-4 min, followed by 600 mg/m² 5-FU IV infusion in 500 ml D_5W over 22 hr. On d two, 200 mg/m² leucovorin IV infusion over 120 min, followed by 400 mg/m² 5-FU IV bolus over 2-4 min, followed by 600 mg/m² 5-FU IV infusion in 500 ml D_5W over 22 hr. Repeat cycle q 2 wk. **Patients with persistent grade 2 neurosensory events:** Reduce dose to 65 mg/m². **Patients with persistent grade 3 neurosensory events:** May need to stop drug. **Patients recovering from grade 3 or 4 GI or hematologic events:** Reduce dose to 65 mg/m². Also reduce dose of 5-FU by 20%.

oxazepam
Apo-Oxazepam*, Novoxapam*, Serax

Benzodiazepine; anxiolytic, sedative-hypnotic
PRC: D; CSS: IV

Available forms
Capsules: 10, 15, 30 mg; *Tablets:* 15 mg

Indications & dosages
➤ *Alcohol withdrawal, severe anxiety*—**Adult:** 15-30 mg PO tid or qid.

---

*Canadian   † Adjust in renal impairment   ‡ Adjust in liver impairment

➤ *Anxiety*—**Adult:** 10-15 mg PO tid or qid. **Elderly:** 10 mg tid, increase to 15 mg tid or qid prn.

oxcarbazepine
Trileptal

Carboxamide derivative; antiepileptic
PRC: C

Available forms
Oral suspension: 60 mg/ml; 300 mg/5 ml; *Tablets (film-coated):* 150, 300, 600 mg

Indications & dosages
➤ *Adjunct therapy for partial seizures*—
Adult: Initially, 300 mg PO bid. May increase to 600 mg PO bid in wkly increments of ≤ 600 mg/d. **Child 4-16 yr:** Initially 8-10 mg/kg/d PO divided bid; max, 600 mg/d divided bid. Increase to target maintenance dose over 2 wk. For patient 20-29 kg, target maintenance dose is 900 mg/d divided bid. For patient > 29-39 kg, target maintenance dose is 1,200 mg/d divided bid. For patient > 39 kg, target maintenance dose is 1,800 mg/d divided bid.†
➤ *Conversion to monotherapy for partial seizures*—**Adult:** 300 mg PO bid while simultaneously reducing the dose of other antiepileptics over 3-6 wk until completely withdrawn. Increase oxcarbazepine by max 600 mg/d q wk over 2-4 wk to 2,400 mg/d divided bid. **Child 4-16 yr:** 8-10 mg/kg/d PO divided bid while simultaneously reducing the dose of other antiepileptics over 3-6 wk until completely withdrawn. Increase oxcarbazepine by max 10 mg/kg/d at wkly intervals.†

➤ *Monotherapy for partial seizures*—
Adult: 300 mg PO bid. Increase by 300 mg/d q 3 d to 1,200 mg/d divided bid. **Child 4-16 yr:** 8-10 mg/kg/d PO divided bid; increase by 5 mg/kg/d q 3rd d to the recommended daily dosage range as follows: If patient weighs 20 kg, 600-900 mg/d; 25 kg, 900-1,200 mg/d; 30 kg, 900-1,200 mg/d; 35 kg, 900-1,500 mg/d; 40 kg, 900-1,500 mg/d; 45 kg, 1,200-1,500 mg/d; 50 kg, 1,200-1,800 mg/d; 55 kg, 1,200-1,800 mg/d; 60 kg, 1,200-2,100 mg/d; 65 kg, 1,200-2,100 mg/d; 70 kg, 1,500-2,100 mg/d.†

oxycodone hydrochloride
OxyContin, OxyFAST, OxyIR, Roxicodone, Roxicodone Intensol, Supeudol*

Opioid; analgesic
PRC: B; CSS: II

Available forms
Capsules: 5 mg; *Oral solution:* 5, 20 mg/ml (concentrate); *Suppository*:* 10, 20 mg; *Tablets:* 5, 15, 30 mg; *Tablets (controlled-release):* 10, 20, 40, 80 mg

Indications & dosages
➤ *Pain*—**Adult:** 10-30 mg PO q 4 hr (5 mg PO q 6 hr for Oxy IR, OxyFAST, and immediate-release capsules). Or, 10-40 mg PR tid or qid. Or, 10 mg controlled-release q 12 hr initially in patients who haven't been taking opioids.

oxytocin, synthetic injection
Pitocin

Exogenous hormone; oxytocic, lactation stimulant
PRC: NR

Available forms
Injection: 10 units/ml

Indications & dosages
➤ *Induction, stimulation of labor*—**Woman:** 10 units added to 1 L D_5W or NSS IV infusion at 1-2 milliunits/min. Increase in increments of ≤ 1-2 milliunits/min q 15-30 min.
➤ *Postpartum bleeding*—**Woman:** 10-40 units added to 1 L D_5W or NSS infusion at 20-40 milliunits/min; 1 ml (10 units) may be given IM after placenta delivery.
➤ *Incomplete or inevitable abortion*—**Woman:** 10 units IV in 500 ml NSS or D_5NSS at 10-20 milliunits/min.

paclitaxel
Taxol

Antimicrotubule drug; antineoplastic
PRC: D

Available forms
Injection: 6 mg/ml

Indications & dosages
➤ *Advanced ovarian CA*—**Adult (previously untreated):** 175 mg/m² IV over 3 hr q 3 wk followed by cisplatin 75 mg/m²; or, 135 mg/m² IV over 24 hr with cisplatin

75 mg/m² q 3 wk. Don't repeat until neutrophil count ≥ 1,500 cells/mm³ and platelet count ≥ 100,000 cells/mm³.‡
Adult (previously treated): 135 or 175 mg/m² IV over 3 hr q 3 wk. Don't repeat until neutrophil count ≥ 1,500 cells/mm³ and platelet count ≥ 100,000 cells/mm³.‡
➤ *Breast CA after failure of combination chemo for metastatic disease or relapse within 6 mo of adjuvant chemo (prior treatment should have included an anthracycline unless contraindicated); adjuvant treatment of node-positive breast CA, given sequentially to standard combination chemo containing doxorubicin*—**Adult:** 175 mg/m² IV over 3 hr q 3 wk. Don't repeat until neutrophil count ≥ 1,500 cells/mm³ and platelet count ≥ 100,000 cells/mm³.‡
➤ *AIDS-related Kaposi's sarcoma*—**Adult:** 135 mg/m² IV over 3 hr q 3 wk or 100 mg/m² IV over 3 hr q 2 wk. Don't repeat until neutrophil count ≥ 1,000 cells/mm³.‡
➤ *Initial treatment of advanced non–small-cell lung CA for patient who isn't candidate for curative surgery or radiation*—**Adult:** 135 mg/m² IV over 24 hr or 175 mg/m² IV over 3 hr. Follow with cisplatin 75 mg/m² or 80 mg/m², respectively. Repeat q 3 wk. Don't repeat until neutrophil count ≥ 1,500 cells/mm³ and platelet count ≥ 100,000 cells/mm³.‡

---

palonosetron hydrochloride
Aloxi

Serotonin (5-HT₃) receptor agonist; antiemetic
PRC: B

Available forms
Injection: 0.25 mg in 5-ml, single-use vial

Indications & dosages
➤ *Prevention of acute and delayed nausea and vomiting from moderately or highly emetogenic chemo*—**Adult:** 0.25 mg IV over 30 sec, 30 min before chemo. Drug is given once per cycle, no more than q 7 d.

pamidronate disodium
Aredia

Diphosphonate, pyrophosphate analogue; antihypercalcemic
PRC: D

Available forms
Powder for injection: 30 mg, 90 mg/vial; *Solution for injection:* 3, 6, 9 mg/ml in 10-ml vials

Indications & dosages
➤ *Hypercalcemia in CA*—**Patient with albumin-corrected serum calcium (CCa) 12-13.5 mg/dl:** 60-90 mg IV over 2-24 hr.† **Patient with CCa > 13.5 mg/dl:** 90 mg IV over 24 hr ≥ 7 d before retreatment.†
➤ *Paget's disease*—**Adult:** 30 mg IV over 4 hr × 3 d. Repeat prn.†

➤ *Osteolytic bone lesions of multiple myeloma*—**Adult:** 90 mg IV over 4 hr q 4 wk.†
➤ *Osteolytic bone lesions of breast CA*—**Adult:** 90 mg IV over 2 hr q 3-4 wk.†

pantoprazole sodium
Protonix, Protonix I.V.

Substituted benzimidazole; gastric acid suppressant
PRC: B

Available forms
Injection: 40 mg; *Tablets (delayed-release):* 20, 40 mg

Indications & dosages
➤ *Esophagitis from GERD*—**Adult:** 40 mg PO daily × ≤ 8 wk; continue another 8 wk prn. If oral therapy is interrupted, may give 40 mg IV daily × 7-10 d.
➤ *Short-term treatment of GERD associated with history of erosive esophagitis*—**Adult:** 40 mg IV daily × 7-10 d. Switch to PO form when tolerated.
➤ *Long-term maintenance of healing erosive esophagitis in patients with GERD*—**Adult:** 40 mg PO daily.
➤ *Pathological hypersecretory conditions, including Zollinger-Ellison syndrome*—**Adult:** Individualize dosage. For short-term treatment, usual dose is 80 mg IV q 12 hr. For those needing a higher dose, 80 mg q 8 hr is expected to maintain acid output less than 10 mEq/hr. Max 240 mg/d. For long-term treatment, usual starting dose is 40 mg PO bid. Max 240 mg/d.

---

§ Adjust in immunocompromised patients　　　¶ Adjust in debilitated patients

paroxetine hydrochloride
Paxil, Paxil CR

SSRI; antidepressant
PRC: C

Available forms
Oral suspension: 10 mg/5 ml; *Tablets:* 10, 20, 30, 40 mg; *Tablets (controlled-release):* 12.5, 25, 37.5 mg

Indications & dosages
➤ *Depression*—**Adult:** 20 mg PO q am. Increase by 10 mg/d at intervals of 1 wk prn to max 50 mg daily. Or, give 25 mg/d (controlled-release); increase prn by 12.5 mg at intervals of at least 1 wk; max 62.5 mg/d.¶ **Elderly:** 10 mg PO q am. Increase 10 mg/d at intervals of 1 wk prn to max 40 mg daily. Or, 12.5 mg/d (controlled-release); may increase prn to max 50 mg/d.†,‡,¶
➤ *Generalized anxiety disorders, post-traumatic stress disorder*—**Adult:** 20 mg PO daily. Increase by 10 mg/d q wk. Max 50 mg/d.†,‡
➤ *Panic disorder*—**Adult:** 10 mg/d. Increase 10 mg/wk prn. Max 60 mg/d. Or, 12.5 mg PO daily (controlled-release); may increase prn by 12.5 mg/wk to max 75 mg/d.†,‡ **Elderly:** 10 mg PO daily. Increase prn to max 40 mg/d. Or, 12.5 mg/d (controlled-release); may increase prn to max 50 mg/d.†,‡,¶
➤ *OCD, social anxiety disorder*—**Adult:** 20 mg PO daily in am. Range 20-60 mg/d.†,‡ **Elderly:** 10 mg PO daily. Increase prn; max 40 mg/d.
➤ *PMDD*—**Woman:** 12.5 mg controlled-release PO daily in am; max 25 mg/d. May

be taken either daily or just during luteal phase of menstrual cycle.†,‡,¶
➤ *Social anxiety disorder*—**Adult:** 12.5 mg (controlled-release) PO daily in am; increase at wkly intervals in increments of 12.5 mg/d, up to max 37.5 mg daily. †,‡,¶

pegfilgrastim
Neulasta

Colony-stimulating factor; neutrophil-growth stimulator
PRC: C

Available forms
Injection: 6 mg/0.6 ml syringes

Indications & dosages
➤ *Prevent infection during myelosuppressive anticancer therapy for non-myeloid malignancies*—**Adult:** 6 mg SC once/chemo cycle. Don't give 14 d before to 24 hr after cytotoxic chemo.

peginterferon alfa-2a
Pegasys

Biological response modifier; antiviral
PRC: C

Available forms
Injection: 180 mcg/0.5 ml

Indications & dosages
➤ *Chronic hepatitis C with compensated hepatic disease in patients not previously treated with interferon alfa*—**Adult:** 180 mcg SC in abdomen or thigh q wk × 48 wk. **Patients with moderate adverse**

---

reactions: Decrease to 135 mcg SC q wk. **Patients with severe adverse reactions:** Decrease to 90 mcg SC q wk. **Patients with hematological reactions and neutrophil count < 750 cells/mm³:** Reduce dose to 135 mcg SC q wk. **Patients with hematological reactions and absolute neutrophil count (ANC) < 500 cells/mm³:** Stop drug until ANC > 1,000 cells/mm³; restart at 90 mcg SC q wk. If platelet count is < 50,000 cells/mm³, reduce dose to 90 mcg SC q wk; stop drug if platelet count goes below 25,000 cells/mm³.†,‡

penicillin G benzathine
Bicillin L-A, Permapen

Natural PCN; antibiotic
PRC: B

Available forms
Injection: 300,000, 600,000 units/ml; 1.2 million units/2 ml; 2.4 million units/ 4 ml

Indications & dosages
➤ *Congenital syphilis*—**Child < 2 yr:** 50,000 units/kg IM × 1 dose.
➤ *Group A strep upper respiratory tract infection*—**Adult:** 1.2 million units IM × 1 dose. **Older child ≥ 27 kg:** 900,000 units IM × 1 dose. **Infant, child < 27 kg:** 300,000-600,000 units IM × 1 dose.
➤ *Prophylaxis of post-strep rheumatic fever*—**Adult, child:** 1.2 million units IM q mo or 600,000 units 2 times/mo.
➤ *Syphilis*—**Adult:** 2.4 million units IM × 1 dose (if duration of infection < 1 yr); or, q wk × 3 wk (if duration of infection > 1 yr).

penicillin G potassium
Pfizerpen

Natural PCN; antibiotic
PRC: B

Available forms
Injection: 1, 2, 3, 5, 20 million units

Indications & dosages
➤ *Systemic infection*—**Adult, child ≥ 12 yr:** 1.2-24 million units IM or IV daily in divided doses q 4 hr.† **Child < 12 yr:** 25,000-400,000 units/kg IM or IV daily in divided doses q 4 hr.†
➤ *Anthrax*—**Adult:** 5-20 million units IV daily in divided doses q 4-6 hr × ≥ 14 d after symptoms subside.† **Child:** 100,000-150,000 units/kg/d IV in divided doses q 4-6 hr × ≥ 14 d after symptoms subside.†

penicillin G procaine

Natural PCN; antibiotic
PRC: B

Available forms
Injection: 600,000, 1.2 million units/ml

Indications & dosages
➤ *Systemic infection*—**Adult:** 600,000-1.2 million units IM daily in 1 dose. **Child > 1 mo:** 25,000-50,000 units/kg IM daily in 1 dose.
➤ *Gonorrhea*—**Adult, child > 12 yr:** 1 g probenecid PO; after 30 min, 4.8 million units IM, divided between 2 sites.

---

§ Adjust in immunocompromised patients ¶ Adjust in debilitated patients

➤ *Pneumococcal pneumonia*—**Adult, child > 12 yr:** 600,000-1.2 million units IM daily × 7-10 d.
➤ *Anthrax, including inhalation anthrax (post-exposure)*—**Adult:** 1.2 million units IM q 12 hr. **Child:** 25,000 units/kg IM (max 1,200,000 units) q 12 hr.
➤ *Cutaneous anthrax*—**Adult:** 600,000-1 million units IM daily.

penicillin G sodium
Crystapen*

Natural PCN; antibiotic
PRC: B

Available forms
Injection: 5 million–unit vial

Indications & dosages
➤ *Systemic infection*—**Adult, child ≥ 12 yr:** 1.2-24 million units daily IM or IV in divided doses q 4-6 hr.† **Child < 12 yr:** 25,000-400,000 units/kg IM or IV in divided doses q 4-6 hr.†

pentoxifylline
Trental

Xanthine derivative; anti-claudication drug
PRC: C

Available forms
Tablets (controlled-release): 400 mg; *Tablets (extended-release):* 400 mg

Indications & dosages
➤ *Intermittent claudication*—**Adult:** 400 mg PO tid with meals. May decrease to 400 mg bid if adverse reactions occur.

pergolide mesylate
Permax

Dopaminergic agonist; antiparkinsonian
PRC: B

Available forms
Tablets: 0.05, 0.25, 1 mg

Indications & dosages
➤ *Parkinson's disease*—**Adult:** 0.05 mg PO daily for 1st 2 d; then increase to 0.1-0.15 mg q 3rd d over 12 d. Then increase 0.25 mg q 3rd d prn until optimum response is achieved. Give in divided doses tid.

perphenazine
Apo-Perphenazine*, PMS Perphenazine*, Trilafon, Trilafon Concentrate

Phenothiazine (piperazine derivative); antipsychotic, antiemetic
PRC: C

Available forms
Injection: 5 mg/ml; *Oral concentration:* 16 mg/5 ml; *Syrup:* 2 mg/5 ml*; *Tablets:* 2, 4, 8, 16 mg

Indications & dosages
➤ *Psychosis in non-hospitalized patient*—**Adult, child > 12 yr:** 4-8 mg PO tid; reduce ASAP to lowest effective dose.
➤ *Psychosis in hospitalized patient*—**Adult, child > 12 yr:** 8-16 mg PO bid-qid; increase to 64 mg/d prn. Or, 5-10 mg IM q 6 hr prn. Max 30 mg.

➤ *Nausea, vomiting*—**Adult:** 8-16 mg PO daily in divided doses to max 24 mg. Or, 5-10 mg IM prn. May give IV; dilute to 0.5 mg/ml with NSS. Max, 5 mg.

phenazopyridine hydrochloride (phenylazo diamino pyridine hydrochloride)
Azo-Standard, Baridium, Geridium, Phenazo*, Prodium, Pyridiate, Pyridium, Pyridium Plus, Urodine, Urogesic

Azo dye; urinary tract analgesic
PRC: B

Available forms
Tablets: 95, 97, 97.2, 100, 150, 200 mg

Indications & dosages
➤ *Pain with urinary tract irritation or UTI*—**Adult:** 200 mg PO tid pc × 2 d. **Child:** 12 mg/kg PO daily in 3 equal doses pc × 2 d.

phenobarbital
Ancalixir*, Barbita, Solfoton

phenobarbital sodium
Luminal Sodium

Barbiturate; anticonvulsant, sedative-hypnotic
PRC: D; CSS: IV

Available forms
Capsules: 16 mg; *Elixir:* 15, 20 mg/5 ml; *Injection:* 30, 60, 65, 130 mg/ml; *Tablets:* 15, 16, 30, 60, 90, 100 mg

Indications & dosages
➤ *Epilepsy, febrile seizures*—**Adult:** 60-200 mg PO daily in divided doses tid or in 1 dose hs. **Child:** 3-6 mg/kg PO daily divided q 12 hr.
➤ *Status epilepticus*—**Adult:** 200-600 mg IV. **Child:** 100-400 mg IV.
➤ *Sedation*—**Adult:** 30-120 mg PO daily in 2-3 divided doses. **Child:** 3-5 mg/kg PO daily in divided doses tid.
➤ *Preop sedation*—**Adult:** 100-200 mg IM 60-90 min preop. **Child:** 16-100 mg IM or 1-3 mg/kg IV, IM, or PO 60-90 min preop.

phenylephrine hydrochloride
Neo-Synephrine

Adrenergic; vasoconstrictor
PRC: C

Available forms
Injection: 10 mg/ml

Indications & dosages
➤ *Hypotension*—**Adult:** 2-5 mg SC or IM; repeat in 1-2 hr prn. Or, 0.1-0.5 mg slow IV; repeat in 10-15 min. **Child:** 0.1 mg/kg IM or SC; repeat in 1-2 hr prn.
➤ *Severe hypotension and shock*—**Adult:** 10 mg in 250-500 ml D_5W or NSS. Start infusion at 100-180 mcg/min; decrease to 40-60 mcg/min when BP is stable.

---

§ Adjust in immunocompromised patients   ¶ Adjust in debilitated patients

phenytoin (diphenylhydantoin)
Dilantin-125, Dilantin Infatabs

phenytoin sodium (prompt)
Dilantin

phenytoin sodium (extended)
Dilantin Kapseals, Phenytek

Hydantoin derivative; anticonvulsant
PRC: NR

Available forms
phenytoin *Oral suspension:* 125 mg/5 ml; *Tablets (chewable):* 50 mg; **sodium (prompt)** *Capsules:* 100 mg (92-mg base); *Injection:* 50 mg/ml (46-mg base); **sodium (extended)** *Capsules:* 30 mg (27.6-mg base), 100 mg (92-mg base), 200 mg (184-mg base), 300 mg (276-mg base)

Indications & dosages
➤ *Seizures*—**Adult:** 100 mg PO tid, increase 100 mg PO q 2-4 wk prn. **Child:** 5 mg/kg or 250 mg/m² PO divided bid or tid. Max 300 mg/d.
➤ *Loading dose*—**Adult:** 1 g PO divided into 3 doses given at 2-hr intervals. Or, 10-15 mg/kg IV at rate not > 50 mg/min. **Child:** 5 mg/kg/d PO in 2 or 3 equally divided doses with later dose individualized to max 300 mg/d.
➤ *Status epilepticus*—**Adult:** Loading dose 10-15 mg/kg IV at rate not > 50 mg/min; then maintenance 100 mg PO or IV q 6-8 hr. **Child:** Loading dose 15-20 mg/kg

IV at rate ≤ 1-3 mg/kg/min; then individualize maintenance doses.

phytonadione (vitamin K₁)
Mephyton

Vitamin K; blood coagulation modifier
PRC: C

Available forms
Injection (aqueous colloidal solution): 2, 10 mg/ml; *Injection (aqueous dispersion):* 2, 10 mg/ml; *Tablets:* 5 mg

Indications & dosages
➤ *Hypoprothrombinemia from vitamin K malabsorption, drug treatment, excessive vitamin A dose*—**Adult:** 2.5-10 mg PO, SC, or IM; repeat and increase up to 50 mg. **Infant:** 2 mg PO, IM, or SC. **Child:** 5-10 mg PO, IM, or SC.
➤ *Hypoprothrombinemia secondary to oral anticoagulants*—**Adult:** 2.5-10 mg PO, SC, or IM. In emergency, 10-50 mg slow IV at a rate not > 1 mg/min; repeat q 4 hr prn.

pilocarpine hydrochloride
Adsorbocarpine, Isopto Carpine, Miocarpine*, Pilocar

pilocarpine nitrate
Pilagan, P.V. Carpine Liquifilm

Cholinergic agonist; miotic
PRC: C

Available forms
hydrochloride *Ophthalmic gel:* 4%; *Ophthalmic solution:* 0.25, 0.5, 1, 2, 3, 4, 5,

---

6, 8, 10%; **nitrate** *Ophthalmic solution:* 1, 2, 4%

Indications & dosages
➤ *Open-angle glaucoma*—**Adult, child:** 1 or 2 drops up to qid, or 1-cm ribbon of 4% gel q hs.
➤ *Acute angle-closure glaucoma*—**Adult, child:** 1 drop 2% solution q 5-10 min × 3-6 doses; then 1 drop q 1-3 hr until pressure controlled.
➤ *Mydriasis*—**Adult, child:** 1 drop 1% solution.

pimecrolimus
Elidel

Topical immunomodulator; topical skin product
PRC: C

Available forms
Cream: 1% in 15-, 30-, and 100-g tubes

Indications & dosages
➤ *Mild-to-moderate atopic dermatitis in non-immunocompromised patients, in whom conventional therapies are inadequate or contraindicated*—**Adult, child ≥ 2 yr:** Thin layer on affected skin bid; rub in gently and completely.

pioglitazone hydrochloride
Actos

Thiazolidinedione; antidiabetic
PRC: C

Available forms
Tablets: 15, 30, 45 mg

Indications & dosages
➤ *Type 2 DM*—**Adult:** 15 or 30 mg PO daily. Increase dose prn; max 45 mg/d. In combination therapy, max 30 mg/d.

piperacillin sodium and tazobactam sodium
Zosyn

Extended-spectrum PCN, beta-lactamase inhibitor; antibiotic
PRC: B

Available forms
Powder for injection: 2, 3, 4 g piperacillin and 0.25, 0.375, 0.5 g tazobactam/vial, respectively

Indications & dosages
➤ *Appendicitis; peritonitis; skin, skin-structure infection; postpartum endometritis; PID; community-acquired pneumonia*—**Adult:** 3 g piperacillin and 0.375 g tazobactam IV q 6 hr × 7-10 d.†
➤ *Nosocomial pneumonia*—**Adult:** 4 g piperacillin and 0.5 g tazobactam IV q 6 hr given with an aminoglycoside.†

potassium chloride
K+10, Kaochlor 10%, K-Dur, Klor-Con, K-Lyte Cl, K-Tab, Slow-K, Ten-K

Potassium (K+) supplement; therapeutic agent for electrolyte balance
PRC: C

Available forms
Capsules (controlled-release): 8, 10 mEq; *Injection concentration:* 1.5, 2 mEq/ml; *Injection for IV infusion:* 0.1, 0.2, 0.3,

§ Adjust in immunocompromised patients　　　　¶ Adjust in debilitated patients

0.4 mEq/ml; *PO liquid:* 20, 30, 40 mEq/
15 ml; *Powder for PO use:* 15, 20,
25 mEq/packet; *Tablets (controlled-release):* 6.7, 8, 10, 20 mEq; *Tablets
(extended-release):* 8, 10 mEq

Indications & dosages

➤ *To prevent hypokalemia*—**Adult, child:**
16-24 mEq PO daily divided; adjust prn.
➤ *Hypokalemia*—**Adult, child:** 40-
100 mEq PO daily divided bid-qid. Use
IV form when PO is not feasible. Max IV
dose, 20 mEq/hr (concentration of
40 mEq/L). Max, 150 mEq PO daily for
adult; 3 mEq/kg PO daily for child.
➤ *Severe hypokalemia*—**Adult, child:**
Concentration should be < 80 mEq/L and
given at ≤ 40 mEq/hr IV. Max, 150 mEq IV
daily for adult; 3 mEq/kg IV daily or
40 mEq/m^2 for child.

potassium gluconate
Kaon, Kaylixir, K-G Elixir

*Potassium supplement; therapeutic agent
for electrolyte balance*
PRC: C

Available forms

Liq: 20 mEq/15 ml; *Tablets:* 500, 595 mg
(83.45 mg and 99 mg potassium, respectively)

Indications & dosages

➤ *Hypokalemia*—**Adult:** 40-100 mEq PO
daily divided bid-qid; 20 mEq daily for
prevention. Adjust prn.

pramipexole
dihydrochloride
Mirapex

Non-ergot dopamine agonist; anti-parkinsonian
PRC: C

Available forms

Tablets: 0.125, 0.25, 1, 1.5 mg

Indications & dosages

➤ *Parkinson's disease*—**Adult:** 0.375 mg
PO daily in divided doses tid; increase q
5-7 d. Maintenance, 1.5-4.5 mg/d in 3 divided doses. †

pravastatin sodium
(eptastatin)
Pravachol

HMG-CoA reductase inhibitor; antilipemic
PRC: X

Available forms

Tablets: 10, 20, 40, 80 mg

Indications & dosages

➤ *To prevent coronary events; hyperlipidemia*—**Adult:** 40 mg PO daily at same
time each d. Adjust dosage q 4 wk prn;
max 80 mg/d.†, ‡, §
➤ *Heterozygous familial hypercholesterolemia*—**Child 14-18 yr:** 40 mg PO daily.
Child 8-13 yr: 20 mg PO daily.†,‡,§

---

prazosin hydrochloride
Minipress

Alpha blocker; antihypertensive
PRC: C

Available forms
Capsules: 1, 2, 5 mg

Indications & dosages
➤ *HTN*—**Adult:** PO test dose 1 mg hs. Then 1 mg PO bid or tid. Increase slowly. Max, 20 mg/d. Maintenance, 6-15 mg/d divided tid.

prednisolone
Delta-Cortef, Prelone

prednisolone acetate
Cotolone, Key-Pred 25, Predalone 50, Predcor-50

prednisolone sodium phosphate
Hydeltrasol, Key-Pred SP, Orapred, Pediapred

prednisolone tebutate
Nor-Pred TBA, Predate TBA, Predcor-TBA, Prednisol TBA

Glucocorticoid; anti-inflammatory, immunosuppressant
PRC: C

Available forms
prednisolone *Syrup:* 5, 15 mg/5 ml; *Tablets:* 5 mg; **acetate** *Injection:* 25, 50 mg/ml; **sodium phosphate** *Injection:* 20 mg/ml; *Oral solution:* 5, 15 mg/5 ml; **tebutate** *Injection (suspension):* 20 mg/ml

Indications & dosages
➤ *Severe inflammation, modification of body's immune response to disease*—**Adult:** 2.5-15 mg prednisolone PO bid-qid. Or, 2-30 mg prednisolone acetate IM q 12 hr. Or, 5-60 mg prednisolone sodium phosphate IM, IV, or PO daily. Or, 4-40 mg prednisolone tebutate into joints and lesions prn. **Child:** 0.14-2 mg/kg/d PO or 4-60 mg/m^2/d in 4 divided doses. Or, 0.04-0.25 mg/kg or 1.5-7.5 mg/m^2 prednisolone acetate IM daily or bid. Or, 0.14-2 mg/kg/d prednisolone sodium phosphate or 4-60 mg/m^2/d in 3 or 4 divided doses IM, IV, or PO.
➤ *Acute exacerbations of MS*—**Adult:** 200 mg/d prednisolone sodium phosphate PO × 1 wk, followed by 80 mg q other d.
➤ *Nephrotic syndrome*—**Child:** 60 mg/m^2/d prednisolone sodium phosphate PO in 3 divided doses for 4 wk, followed by 4 wk of single-dose alternate-day therapy at 40 mg/m^2/d.
➤ *Uncontrolled asthma in patients taking inhaled corticosteroids and long-acting bronchodilators*—**Child:** 1-2 mg/kg/d prednisolone sodium phosphate PO in single or divided doses. Continue short course, or "burst" therapy, until child achieves peak expiratory flow rate of 80% of his personal best or symptoms resolve, usually 3-10 d.

---

§ Adjust in immunocompromised patients   ¶ Adjust in debilitated patients

prednisone
Liquid Pred, Meticorten, Panasol-S, Prednicen-M, Prednisone Intensol

Adrenocorticoid; anti-inflammatory, immunosuppressant
PRC: C

Available forms
Oral solution: 5 mg/5 ml, 5 mg/ml (concentrate); *Syrup:* 5 mg/5 ml; *Tablets:* 1, 2.5, 5, 10, 20, 50 mg

Indications & dosages
➤ *Inflammation, immunosuppression—* **Adult:** 5-60 mg PO daily in 1-4 divided doses. Give maintenance dose daily or q other d. **Child:** 0.14-2 mg/kg or 4-60 mg/m² PO daily in 4 divided doses.

primidone
Apo-Primidone*, Mysoline, PMS Primidone*, Sertan*

Barbiturate analogue; anticonvulsant
PRC: NR

Available forms
Oral suspension: 250 mg/5 ml; *Tablets:* 50, 250 mg

Indications & dosages
➤ *Seizures—***Adult, child ≥ 8 yr:** 100-125 mg PO hs on d 1-3; 100-125 mg PO bid on d 4-6; 100-125 mg PO tid on d 7-9; then 250 mg PO tid. Increase to 250 mg qid prn. Max, 2 g/d in divided doses. **Child < 8 yr:** 50 mg PO hs × 3 d; then 50 mg PO bid on d 4-6, 100 mg PO bid on d 7-9; then 125-250 mg PO tid.

probenecid
Benemid, Benuryl*

Sulfonamide derivative; uricosuric
PRC: NR

Available forms
Tablets: 500 mg

Indications & dosages
➤ *Gonorrhea—***Adult:** 1 g PO with 3.5 g ampicillin PO; or 1 g PO 30 min before dose of 4.8 million units aqueous PCN G procaine IM; inject at 2 different sites.
➤ *Hyperuricemia of gout, gouty arthritis—***Adult:** 250 mg PO bid × 1 wk; then 500 mg bid. Max, 2 g/d.
➤ *Prevent RF after cidofovir infusion—* **Adult:** 2 g PO 3 hr before cidofovir infusion; then 1 g PO 2 and 8 hr after infusion.

procainamide hydrochloride
Procanbid, Promine, Pronestyl

Procaine derivative; ventricular and supraventricular antiarrhythmic
PRC: C

Available forms
Capsules: 250, 375, 500 mg; *Injection:* 100, 500 mg/ml; *Tablets:* 250, 375, 500 mg; *Tablets (extended-release):* 250, 500, 750, 1,000 mg

Indications & dosages
➤ *Ventricular arrhythmias—***Adult:** 100 mg slow IV push at a rate ≤ 50 mg/min q 5 min until arrhythmias disappear,

adverse reactions develop, or 500 mg given. Continue infusion of 2-6 mg/min. If arrhythmias recur, repeat bolus and increase infusion rate. Or, 50 mg/kg IM divided q 3-6 hr; for arrhythmias during surgery, 100-500 mg IM. Or, 50 mg/kg/d in divided doses q 3 hr. May divide doses of extended-release tablets q 6 hr and Procanbid q 12 hr.†

prochlorperazine
Compazine, PMS Prochlorperazine*

prochlorperazine edisylate
Compazine, Cotranzine, Ultrazine-10

prochlorperazine maleate
Compazine, PMS Prochlorperazine*, Stemetil*

Phenothiazine (piperazine derivative); antipsychotic, antiemetic, anxiolytic
PRC: NR

Available forms
prochlorperazine *Injection:* 5 mg/ml; *Suppository:* 2.5, 5, 25 mg; *Tablets:* 5, 10 mg; **edisylate** *Injection:* 5 mg/ml; *Syrup:* 5 mg/5 ml; **maleate** *Capsules (extended-release):* 10, 15, 30 mg; *Tablets:* 5, 10, 25 mg

Indications & dosages
➤ *Preop nausea*—**Adult:** 5-10 mg IM 1-2 hr before anesthesia; may repeat once in 30 min. Or, 5-10 mg IV 15-30 min before anesthesia; repeat once prn.
➤ *Nausea, vomiting*—**Adult:** 5-10 mg PO tid or qid; 25 mg PR bid; 5-10 mg IM, repeat q 3-4 hr prn. Or, 2.5-10 mg IV at max

rate 5 mg/min. **Child 9-13 kg:** 2.5 mg PO or PR daily or bid. Or, 0.132 mg/kg IM. **Child 14-17 kg:** 2.5 mg PO or PR bid or tid. Or, 0.132 mg/kg deep IM. **Child 18-39 kg:** 2.5 mg PO or PR tid; or 5 mg PO or PR bid. Or, 0.132 mg/kg deep IM.
➤ *Psychotic disorders*—**Adult:** 5-10 mg PO tid or qid. **Child 2-12 yr:** 2.5 mg PO or PR bid or tid. Max 10 mg on d 1. Increase dose prn. Child 2-10 yr, max 25 mg/d.
➤ *Anxiety*—**Adult:** 5-10 mg deep IM q 3-4hr; max 20 mg/d. Treat ≤ 12 wk. Or, 5-10 mg PO tid-qid. Or, 15 mg extended-release capsules daily or 10 mg extended-release capsules q 12 hr.

promethazine hydrochloride
Anergan 50, Phenergan

Phenothiazine derivative; antiemetic, antivertigo drug, H_1-receptor antagonist, adjunct to analgesics, sedative
PRC: C

Available forms
Injection: 25, 50 mg/ml; *Suppository:* 12.5, 25, 50 mg; *Syrup:* 6.25 mg/5 ml; *Tablets:* 12.5, 25, 50 mg

Indications & dosages
➤ *Motion sickness*—**Adult:** 25 mg PO bid. **Child:** 12.5-25 mg PO, IM, or PR bid.
➤ *Nausea*—**Adult:** 12.5-25 mg PO, IM, or PR q 4-6 hr prn. **Child:** 12.5-25 mg IM or PR q 4-6 hr prn.
➤ *Rhinitis, allergy symptoms*—**Adult:** 12.5 mg PO qid; or 25 mg PO hs. **Child:** 6.25-12.5 mg PO tid or 25 mg PO or PR hs.

§ Adjust in immunocompromised patients   ¶ Adjust in debilitated patients

➤ *Sedation*—**Adult:** 25-50 mg PO or IM hs or prn. **Child:** 12.5-25 mg PO, IM, or PR hs.
➤ *Preop or postop sedation, adjunct to analgesics*—**Adult:** 25-50 mg IM, IV, or PO. **Child:** 12.5-25 mg IM, IV, or PO.

propafenone hydrochloride
Rythmol

Sodium channel antagonist; anti-arrhythmic
PRC: C

Available forms
Tablets: 150, 225, 300 mg

Indications & dosages
➤ *Ventricular arrhythmias*—**Adult:** 150 mg PO q 8 hr. May increase dose q 3 or 4 d; max, 225 mg q 8 hr. If needed, 300 mg q 8 hr. Max, 900 mg/d.

propofol
Diprivan

Phenol derivative; anesthetic
PRC: B

Available forms
Injection: 10 mg/ml in 20-ml amp; 50-ml prefilled syringes; 50-, 100-ml infusion vials

Indications & dosages
➤ *Sedation in mechanically ventilated patient*—**Adult:** 5 mcg/kg/min × 5 min. Increase rate q 5-10 min in 5-10 mcg/kg/min increments prn. Usual maintenance infusion rate, 5-50 mcg/kg/min.

propoxyphene hydrochloride
Darvon, 692*, Darvon Pulvules

propoxyphene napsylate
Darvon-N

Opioid analgesic; opioid analgesic
PRC: C; CSS IV

Available forms
hydrochloride *Capsules:* 65 mg; **napsylate** *Oral suspension:* 50 mg/5 ml; *Tablets (film-coated):* 100 mg

Indications & dosages
➤ *Pain*—**Adult:** 65 mg hydrochloride PO q 4 hr prn. Max, 390 mg/d. Or, 100 mg napsylate PO q 4 hr prn. Max, 600 mg/d.

propranolol hydrochloride
Detensol*, Inderal, Inderal LA, InnoPran XL, Novopranol*

Beta blocker; antihypertensive, antianginal, antiarrhythmic, adjunctive treatment for MI
PRC: C

Available forms
Capsules (extended-release): 60, 80, 120, 160 mg; *Injection:* 1 mg/ml; *Oral solution:* 20, 40 mg/5 ml, 80 mg/ml (concentrate); *Tablets:* 10, 20, 40, 60, 80 mg

Indications & dosages
➤ *Angina*—**Adult:** Total daily dose 80-320 mg PO bid-qid; or one 80-mg extended-release capsule daily. Increase q 7-10 d.

➤ *MI*—**Adult:** 180-240 mg PO tid or qid 5-21 d post-MI.

➤ *Supraventricular, ventricular arrhythmias; tachyarrhythmias during anesthesia*—**Adult:** 0.5-3 mg IV push × ≤ 1 mg/min. After 3 mg, next dose in 2 min; additional doses in > 4-hr intervals. Maintenance, 10-30 mg PO tid or qid.

➤ *HTN*—**Adult:** 80 mg PO daily in 2-4 divided doses or extended-release (Inno-Pran XL) q hs. Increase q 3-7 d. Max, 640 mg/d. Maintenance, 160-480 mg/d.

➤ *Essential tremor*—**Adult:** 40 mg PO bid. Maintenance, 120-320 mg/d in 3 divided doses.

➤ *Hypertrophic subaortic stenosis*—**Adult:** 20-40 mg PO tid or qid, or 80-160 mg extended-release capsules in 1 dose/d.

➤ *Pheochromocytoma*—**Adult:** 60 mg PO daily in divided doses with an alpha blocker 3 d preop.

propylthiouracil (PTU)
Propyl-Thyracil*

Thyroid hormone antagonist; antihyperthyroid
PRC: D

Available forms
Tablets: 50 mg

Indications & dosages
➤ *Hyperthyroidism*—**Adult:** 300-450 mg daily in divided doses. Continue until patient is euthyroid, then, maintenance, 100 mg PO once daily divided tid. **Child > 10 yr:** 150-300 mg PO daily in divided doses q 8 hr or 150 mg/m²/d in divided

doses q 8 hr. Continue until patient is euthyroid, then individualize maintenance dose. **Child 6-10 yr:** 50-150 mg PO daily in divided doses q 8 hr. Continue until patient is euthyroid, then individualize maintenance dose. **Neonates:** 5-10 mg/kg/d in divided doses q 8 hr.

➤ *Thyrotoxic crisis*—**Adult:** 200 mg PO q 4-6 hr on d 1. Reduce dose to maintenance level.

protamine sulfate

Antidote; heparin antagonist
PRC: C

Available forms
Injection: 10 mg/ml

Indications & dosages
➤ *Heparin overdose*—**Adult:** Dose based on coagulation studies, usually 1 mg for each 90-115 units heparin. Max, 50 mg.

pseudoephedrine hydrochloride
Cenafed, Decofed, Dimetapp, Efidac/24, Genaphed, PediaCare Infants' Decongestant, Sudafed, Triaminic

pseudoephedrine sulfate
Drixoral 12 Hour Non-Drowsy Formula

Adrenergic; decongestant
PRC: C

Available forms
hydrochloride *Capsules:* 60 mg; *Capsules (liquid gel):* 30 mg; *Oral solution:* 7.5 mg/0.8 ml, 15 mg/5 ml, 30 mg/5 ml; *Tablets:*

---

§ Adjust in immunocompromised patients   ¶ Adjust in debilitated patients

30, 60 mg; Tablets (chewable): 15 mg; Tablets (controlled-release): 240 mg; Tablets (extended-release): 120, 240 mg; **sulfate** Tablets (extended-release): 240 mg

Indications & dosages
➤ *Decongestant*—**Adult, child ≥ 12 yr:** 60 mg PO q 4-6 hr; or 120 mg PO extended-release tablet q 12 hr. Or, 240 mg PO controlled-release tablet daily. Max, 240 mg daily. **Child 6-12 yr:** 30 mg PO q 4-6 hr. Max, 120 mg daily. **Child 2-5 yr:** 15 mg PO q 4-6 hr. Max, 60 mg daily. Or, 4 mg/kg or 125 mg/m^2 PO divided qid.

pyridoxine hydrochloride (vitamin B$_6$)

H_2O-soluble vitamin; nutritional supplement
PRC: A

Available forms
Injection: 100 mg/ml; Tablets: 10, 25, 50, 100, 200, 250, 500 mg; Tablets (extended-release): 200 mg

Indications & dosages
➤ *Dietary vitamin B$_6$ deficiency*—**Adult:** 10-20 mg PO, IM, or IV daily × 3 wk; then 2-5 mg/d as supplement to proper diet.
➤ *Seizures related to vitamin B$_6$ deficiency or dependency*—**Adult, child:** 100 mg IM or IV in 1 dose.
➤ *To prevent isoniazid pyridoxine deficiency*—**Adult:** 10-50 mg PO daily.

➤ *Isoniazid toxicity (> 10 g)*—**Adult:** Give amount equal to isoniazid taken: Generally, 1-4 g IV, then, 1 g IM q 30 min until entire dose is given.

quetiapine fumarate
Seroquel

Dibenzapine derivative; antipsychotic
PRC: C

Available forms
Tablets: 25, 100, 200, 300 mg

Indications & dosages
➤ *Psychotic disorders*—**Adult:** 25 mg PO bid. Increase by 25-50 mg bid or tid on d 2 and 3, as tolerated. Target dose, 300-400 mg daily, divided bid or tid, by d 4. Adjust dose q ≥ 2 d prn. **Elderly:** Lower doses, slow adjustment; carefully monitor in initial dose period. Adjust dose in hypotensive patient.†, ‡
➤ *Acute bipolar mania with lithium or divalproex*—**Adult:** 50 mg PO bid. Increase in increments of 100 mg/d in 2 divided doses up to 200 mg bid on d 4. May increase in increments no > 200 mg/d up to 800 mg/d by d 6. Usual, 400-800 mg daily.†, ‡

quinapril hydrochloride
Accupril

ACE inhibitor; antihypertensive
PRC: C (D, 2nd and 3rd trimesters)

Available forms
Tablets: 5, 10, 20, 40 mg

Indications & dosages

➤ *HTN*—**Adult ≤ 65 yr:** 10 or 20 mg PO daily or 5 mg/d if patient is using diuretic.† **Adult > 65 yr:** Initially 10 mg PO daily; adjust q 2 wk prn.†

➤ *HF*—**Adult:** 5 mg PO bid. Increase at wkly intervals. Max, 20 mg bid.†

quinidine gluconate
Quinate*

quinidine sulfate
Apo-Quinidine*, Cin-Quin, Quinidex Extentabs

Cinchona alkaloid; anti-tachyarrhythmic
PRC: C

Available forms

gluconate *Injection:* 80 mg/ml; *Tablets (extended-release):* 324, 325*; *sulfate Injection:* 200 mg/ml*; *Tablets:* 200, 300 mg; *Tablets (extended-release):* 300 mg

Indications & dosages

➤ *Atrial fibrillation, flutter*—**Adult:** 200 mg PO q 2-3 hr × 5-8 doses; then increase daily. Max, 3-4 g/d.

➤ *PSVT*—**Adult:** 400-600 mg IM or PO q 2-3 hr.

➤ *PAC; PVC; PAT; PVT; maintenance after cardioversion of atrial fibrillation*—**Adult:** Test dose, 200 mg PO or IM; then 200-400 mg sulfate or equivalent base PO q 4-6 hr. Or, 600 mg gluconate IM; then 400 mg q 2 hr prn. Or, 800 mg gluconate in 40 ml D$_5$W IV at 16 mg/min. **Child:** Test dose, 2 mg/kg PO; then 30 mg/kg/24 hr

PO or 900 mg/m²/24 hr PO in 5 divided doses.

quinupristin and dalfopristin
Synercid

Streptogramin; antibiotic
PRC: B

Available forms

Injection: 500 mg/10 ml (150 mg quinupristin, 350 mg dalfopristin)

Indications & dosages

➤ *Vancomycin-resistant* Enterococcus faecium *bacteremia*—**Adult, adolescent ≥ 16 yr:** 7.5 mg/kg IV over 1 hr q 8 hr.

➤ *Skin, skin-structure infection from* Staphylococcus aureus *(methicillin susceptible) or* Streptococcus pyogenes—**Adult, adolescent ≥ 16 yr:** 7.5 mg/kg IV over 1 hr q 12 hr ≥ 7 d.

rabeprazole sodium
Aciphex

Proton pump inhibitor; antiulcerative
PRC: B

Available forms

Tablets (delayed-release): 20 mg

Indications & dosages

➤ *GERD*—**Adult:** 20 mg PO daily × 4-8 wk. May continue another 8 wk prn.

➤ *To maintain healing of GERD*—**Adult:** 20 mg PO daily.

---

§ Adjust in immunocompromised patients   ¶ Adjust in debilitated patients

➤ *Symptomatic GERD, including daytime and nighttime heartburn*—**Adult:** 20 mg PO daily × 4 wk. May continue another 4 wk prn.

➤ *Duodenal ulcers*—**Adult:** 20 mg PO daily in am pc ≤ 4 wk.

➤ *To prevent recurrence of ulcer from* Helicobacter pylori *infection*—20 mg PO bid with amoxicillin 1,000 mg PO bid and clarithromycin 500 mg PO bid × 7 d.

➤ *Hypersecretory conditions (Zollinger-Ellison syndrome)*—**Adult:** 60 mg PO daily; increase prn to 100 mg daily or 60 mg bid.

---

raloxifene hydrochloride
Evista

Selective estrogen receptor modulator; antiosteoporotic
PRC: X

Available forms
Tablets: 60 mg

Indications & dosages
➤ *To prevent osteoporosis*—**Adult:** 60 mg PO daily.

---

ramipril
Altace

ACE inhibitor; antihypertensive
PRC: C (D, 2nd and 3rd trimesters)

Available forms
Capsules: 1.25, 2.5, 5, 10 mg

Indications & dosages
➤ *HTN*—**Adult:** 2.5 mg PO daily for patient not taking diuretic; 1.25 mg PO daily for patient taking diuretic. Increase prn. Maintenance, 2.5-20 mg/d in single dose or divided bid.†

➤ *HF*—**Adult:** 2.5 mg PO bid. If hypotension, decrease to 1.25 mg PO bid. May increase to max 5 mg PO bid prn.†

➤ *To reduce risk of MI, stroke, death from CV causes*—**Adult ≥ 55 yr:** 2.5 mg PO daily × 1 wk, then 5 mg PO daily × 3 wk. Increase to maintenance dose of 10 mg PO daily. For HTN or recent MI patient, divide daily dose.†

---

ranitidine hydrochloride
Apo-Ranitidine*, Zantac, Zantac-C*, Zantac EFFERdose, Zantac 75

H₂-receptor antagonist; antiulcerative
PRC: B

Available forms
Capsules: 150, 300 mg; *Injection:* 1 mg/ml premixed in 50 ml of ½ NSS, 25 mg/ml in 2- and 6-ml vials; *Syrup:* 15 mg/ml; *Tablets:* 75, 150, 300 mg; *Tablets/granules (effervescent):* 150 mg

Indications & dosages
➤ *Duodenal, gastric ulcer; hypersecretory conditions (Zollinger-Ellison syndrome)*—**Adult:** 150 mg PO bid or 300 mg/d hs. Or, 50 mg IV or IM q 6-8 hr. For Zollinger-Ellison syndrome, max 6 g PO daily.†

➤ *Maintenance therapy for duodenal, gastric ulcer*—**Adult:** 150 mg PO hs.†

➤ *GERD*—**Adult:** 150 mg PO bid.†

---

*Canadian   † Adjust in renal impairment   ‡ Adjust in liver impairment

repaglinide
Prandin

Meglitinide; antidiabetic
PRC: C

Available forms
Tablets: 0.5, 1, 2 mg

Indications & dosages
➤ *Type 2 DM, alone or with metformin, rosiglitazone maleate, or pioglitazone HCl*—**Adult not previously treated or with HbA$_{1c}$ < 8%:** 0.5 mg PO up to 30 min each ac.† **Adult previously on glucose-lowering drugs and HbA$_{1c}$ ≥ 8%:** 1-2 mg PO up to 30 min each ac. Range 0.5-4 mg with meals divided bid-qid. Max 16 mg/d.†

rifabutin
Mycobutin

Semisynthetic antimycobacterial; antibiotic
PRC: B

Available forms
Capsules: 150 mg

Indications & dosages
➤ *To prevent disseminated MAC in HIV infection*—**Adult:** 300 mg PO daily in 1 dose or divided bid with food.

rifampin
Rifadin, Rifadin IV, Rimactane, Rofact*

Semisynthetic rifamycin B derivative (macrocyclic antibiotic); antituberculotic
PRC: C

Available forms
Capsules: 150, 300 mg; *Injection:* 600 mg

Indications & dosages
➤ *Pulmonary TB*—**Adult:** 600 mg/d PO or IV 1 hr ac or 2 hr pc. **Child > 5 yr:** 10-20 mg/kg PO or IV daily 1 hr ac or 2 hr pc. Max, 600 mg/d.
➤ *Meningococcal carriers*—**Adult:** 600 mg PO or IV bid × 2 d, or 600 mg/d PO or IV daily × 4 d. **Child 1 mo-12 yr:** 10 mg/kg PO or IV bid × 2 d, ≤ 600 mg/d, or 10-20 mg/kg PO or IV × 4 d. **Neonate:** 5 mg/kg PO or IV bid × 2 d.
➤ *To prevent Haemophilus influenzae type B*—**Adult, child:** 20 mg/kg/d PO × 4 d; max, 600 mg/d.

rifapentine
Priftin

RNA polymerase inhibitor; antituberculotic
PRC: C

Available forms
Tablets (film-coated): 150 mg

Indications & dosages
➤ *Pulmonary TB*—**Adult:** Intensive phase, 600 mg PO 2 times/wk × 2 mo, doses ≥ 72 hr apart. Continuation phase, 600 mg PO q wk × 4 mo.

§ Adjust in immunocompromised patients   ¶ Adjust in debilitated patients

risedronate sodium
Actonel

Bisphosphonate; antiresorptive drug
PRC: C

Available forms
Tablets: 5, 30, 35 mg

Indications & dosages
➤ *To prevent and treat postmenopausal osteoporosis*—**Adult:** 5 mg PO daily or 35-mg tablet q wk ≥ 30 min before 1st food or liq of d. Give while patient is upright with 6-8 oz water.
➤ *To prevent and treat glucocorticoid-induced osteoporosis*—**Adult:** 5 mg PO daily ≥ 30 min before 1st food or liq of d. Give while patient is upright with 6-8 oz water.
➤ *Paget's disease*—**Adult:** 30 mg PO daily × 2 mo. If treatment fails, may repeat ≥ 2 mo after completing 1st treatment.

risperidone
Risperdal, Risperdal Consta, Risperdal M-Tab

Benzisoxazole derivative; antipsychotic
PRC: C

Available forms
Oral solution: 1 mg/ml; *Powder for IM injection:* 25, 37.5, 50 mg; *Tablets:* 0.25, 0.5, 1, 2, 3, 4 mg; *Tablets (orally disintegrating):* 0.5, 1, 2 mg

Indications & dosages
➤ *6-8 wk therapy for schizophrenia*—**Adult:** 1 mg PO bid. Increase by 1 mg bid on d 2 and 3 to target dose of 3 mg bid. Or, 1 mg PO on d 1; 2 mg on d 2; and 4 mg on d 3. Wait at least 1 wk before adjusting dosage further. Adjust doses by 1-2 mg up to 8 mg/d.†.‡.¶
➤ *To delay relapse in 1-2 yr therapy for schizophrenia*—**Adult:** 1 mg PO on d 1; 2 mg on d 2; and 4 mg on d 3. Range 2-8 mg daily.†, ‡, ¶ *Elderly or patients at risk of hypotension:* 0.5 mg PO bid. Increase by 0.5 mg bid. Give increase > 1.5 mg bid at intervals of at least 1 wk. May switch to daily dosing after patient has been using bid regimen for 2-3 d at target dose.
➤ *12 wk therapy for schizophrenia*—**Adult:** Establish tolerance to PO drug before giving IM. 25 mg Risperdal Consta deep IM gluteal injection q 2 wk. Adjust dose ≥ q 4 wk. Max, 50 mg q 2 wk. Continue PO drug for 3 wk after 1st IM injection; then stop PO therapy.†.‡.¶
➤ *Monotherapy or combination therapy with lithium or valproate for the short-term (3 wk) treatment of acute manic or mixed episodes associated with bipolar disorder*—**Adult:** 2-3 mg PO daily. Adjust by 1 mg daily. Dosage range, 1-6 mg daily.†.‡.¶

ritonavir
Norvir

HIV protease inhibitor; antiviral
PRC: B

Available forms
Capsules: 100 mg; *Oral solution:* 80 mg/ml

Indications & dosages
➤ *HIV infection*—**Adult:** 600 mg PO bid ac. If patient is nauseated, give 300 mg bid × 1 d, 400 mg bid × 2 d, 500 mg bid × 1 d, and 600 mg bid thereafter.

rivastigmine tartrate
Exelon

Cholinesterase inhibitor; cholinomimetic
PRC: B

Available forms
Capsules: 1.5, 3, 4.5, 6 mg; *Solution:* 2 mg/ml

Indications & dosages
➤ *Alzheimer's disease*—**Adult:** 1.5 mg PO bid with food. Increase to 3 mg bid after 2 wk, as tolerated; then increase to 4.5 mg bid and 6 mg bid as tolerated after 2 wk on previous dose. Range 6-12 mg/d; max 12 mg/d.

rofecoxib
Vioxx

Cyclooxygenase-2 inhibitor; nonopioid analgesic, anti-inflammatory
PRC: C

Available forms
Oral suspension: 12.5 mg/5 ml, 25 mg/5 ml; *Tablets:* 12.5, 25, 50 mg

Indications & dosages
➤ *OA*—**Adult:** 12.5 mg PO daily; increase prn to max 25 mg daily.
➤ *Pain, primary dysmenorrhea*—**Adult:** 50 mg PO daily prn ≤ 5 d.

➤ *RA*—**Adult:** 25 mg PO daily. Max, 25 mg/d.

ropinirole hydrochloride
Requip

Nonergoline dopamine agonist; antiparkinsonian
PRC: C

Available forms
Tablets: 0.25, 0.5, 1, 2, 5 mg

Indications & dosages
➤ *Parkinson's disease*—**Adult:** 0.25 mg PO tid. Adjust wkly. After wk 4, may increase by 1.5 mg wkly up to 9 mg/d; then increase wkly up to 3 mg/d. Max, 24 mg/d.

rosiglitazone maleate
Avandia

Thiazolidinedione; antidiabetic
PRC: C

Available forms
Tablets: 2, 4, 8 mg

Indications & dosages
➤ *Type 2 DM alone, or with metformin, insulin, or sulfonylureas*—**Adult:** 4 mg PO daily in am or in divided doses bid in am and pm. May increase to 8 mg PO daily or in divided doses bid after 12 wk of therapy. With insulin, use only 4 mg dose.

rosiglitazone maleate and metformin hydrochloride
Avandamet

Thiazolidinedione and biguanide; anti-diabetic
PRC: C

Available forms
Tablets: 1, 2, 4 mg rosiglitazone maleate and 500 mg metformin hydrochloride

Indications & dosages
➤ *Type 2 DM inadequately controlled by metformin or rosiglitazone alone—***Adult:** Give individualized dose bid with meals; dose based on patient's current doses of rosiglitazone or metformin. If taking metformin alone, 2 mg rosiglitazone PO bid, plus dose of metformin already being taken (500 or 1,000 mg PO bid). May increase dose after 8-12 wk. If taking rosiglitazone alone, 500 mg metformin PO bid, plus dose of rosiglitazone already being taken (2 or 4 mg PO bid). May increase dose after 1-2 wk. May increase total daily dose in increments of 4 mg rosiglitazone or 500 mg metformin, or both, up to max daily dose 8 mg/2,000 mg in 2 divided doses. **Elderly:** Initial and maintenance doses should be given cautiously.

rosuvastatin calcium
Crestor

HMG-CoA reductase inhibitor; antilipemic
PRC: X

Available forms
Tablets: 5, 10, 20, 40 mg

Indications & dosages
➤ *With diet, to reduce total cholesterol, LDL, apolipoprotein B (ApoB), non–HDL, and triglyceride (TG) levels, and to increase HDL level in primary hypercholesterolemia (heterozygous familial and nonfamilial) and mixed dyslipidemia (Fredrickson types IIa and IIb); also with diet, to treat elevated TG levels (Fredrickson type IV)—***Adult:** 10 mg PO once daily. May increase prn q 2-4 wk to max 40 mg daily based on lipid levels. For aggressive lipid lowering, starting dosage may be 20 mg daily.†
➤ *With other lipid-lowering therapies, to reduce LDL, ApoB, and total cholesterol levels in homozygous familial hypercholesterolemia—***Adult:** 20 mg PO once daily. Max 40 mg daily.†

salmeterol xinafoate
Serevent Diskus

Selective beta₂-adrenergic agonist; bronchodilator
PRC: C

Available forms
Inhalation powder: 50 mcg/blister

Indications & dosages
➤ *Asthma, to prevent bronchospasm in nocturnal asthma or reversible obstructive airway disease—***Adult, child ≥ 4 yr:** 1 inhalation in am and pm, approximately 12 hr apart.

➤ *COPD, emphysema*—**Adult:** 1 inhalation in am and pm, approximately 12 hr apart.

saquinavir
Fortovase
saquinavir mesylate
Invirase

Protease inhibitor; antiviral
PRC: B

Available forms
saquinavir *Capsules (soft gelatin):* 200 mg; **mesylate** *Capsules (hard gelatin):* 200 mg

Indications & dosages
➤ *HIV infection*—**Adult, child >16 yr:** 1,200 mg (Fortovase) PO tid within 2 hr pc. Or, 1,000 mg (Invirase or Fortovase) bid with 100 mg ritonavir bid.

sargramostim (granulocyte macrophage-colony stimulating factor, GM-CSF)
Leukine, Leukine Liquid

Biological response modifier; colony-stimulating factor
PRC: C

Available forms
Injection: 500 mcg/ml; *Powder for injection:* 250 mcg

Indications & dosages
➤ *To accelerate hematopoiesis after autologous bone marrow transplant*

(BMT)—**Adult:** 250 mcg/m^2/d IV over 2 hr × 21 d starting 2-4 hr after BMT.
➤ *BMT failure, engraftment delay*—**Adult:** 250 mcg/m^2/d IV over 2 hr × 14 d. May repeat dose after 7 d of no treatment.

scopolamine (hyoscine)
Isopto Hyoscine, Scopace, Transderm-Scōp

scopolamine hydrobromide (hyoscine hydrobromide)

Anticholinergic; antimuscarinic, cycloplegic mydriatic
PRC: C

Available forms
scopolamine *Ophthalmic solution:* 0.25%; *Transdermal patch:* 1.5 mg/ 2.5 cm^2 (1 mg/72 hr); **hydrobromide** *Injection:* 0.3, 0.4, 1 mg/ml in 1-ml vials and ampules, 0.86 mg/ml in 0.5-ml ampules; *Tablets (soluble):* 0.4 mg

Indications & dosages
➤ *Cycloplegic refraction*—**Adult:** 1 or 2 drops ophthalmic solution 1 hr before refraction. **Child:** 1 drop ophthalmic solution bid × 2 d before refraction.
➤ *Iritis, uveitis*—**Adult:** 1 or 2 drops ophthalmic solution q d to tid. **Child:** 1 drop q d to tid.
➤ *Delirium, preanesthetic sedation and obstetric amnesia with analgesics*—**Adult:** 0.3-0.65 mg IM, SC, or IV. May repeat 3 or 4 times/d prn. Or, 0.4-0.8 mg PO. **Child:** 0.006 mg/kg IM, SC, IV; max 0.3 mg.

---

§ Adjust in immunocompromised patients   ¶ Adjust in debilitated patients

➤ *Motion sickness*—**Adult:** 1 Transderm-Scōp patch applied to skin behind ear several hr before antiemetic required. Or, 0.25-0.5 mg PO 1 hr before motion. May repeat dose 3 or 4 times/d prn

selegiline hydrochloride
Atapryl, Carbex, Eldepryl, Selpak

MAO-B inhibitor; antiparkinsonian
PRC: C

Available forms
Capsules: 5 mg; *Tablets:* 5 mg

Indications & dosages
➤ *Parkinson's disease*—**Adult:** 10 mg/d PO (5 mg at breakfast and 5 mg at lunch). After 2 or 3 d, slowly decrease levodopa and carbidopa dose.

sertaconazole nitrate
Ertaczo

Imidazole derivative; topical antifungal
PRC: C

Available forms
Topical cream: 2%, in 15-and 30 g tubes

Indications & dosages
➤ *Interdigital tinea pedis caused by* Trichophyton rubrum, T. mentagrophytes, *and* Epidermophyton floccosum—**Immunocompetent adult or child ≥ 12 yr:** Apply cream bid to affected areas between toes and to surrounding healthy areas × 4 wk.

sertraline hydrochloride
Zoloft

SSRI; antidepressant
PRC: B

Available forms
Oral concentrate: 20 mg/ml; *Tablets:* 25, 50, 100 mg

Indications & dosages
➤ *Depression*—**Adult:** 50 mg/d PO; adjust dose prn at ≥ 1-wk intervals.
➤ *OCD*—**Adult:** 50 mg/d PO. Max, 200 mg/d. Adjust dose at ≥ 1-wk intervals.
➤ *Posttraumatic stress disorder, social anxiety disorder*—**Adult:** 25 mg PO daily. Increase to 50 mg PO daily after 1 wk. Adjust dose q wk to max 200 mg/d. Maintain patient on lowest effective dose.‡
➤ *PMDD*—**Adult:** 50 mg PO daily continuously or only during luteal phase. May increase at 50 mg increments/menstrual cycle up to 150 mg daily for continuous dosing or 100 mg daily for luteal phase dosing. If using 100 mg daily for luteal phase dosing, begin with 50 mg daily adjustment step × 3 d, then increase to 100 mg on d 4 and for remainder of luteal phase.

sibutramine hydrochloride monohydrate
Meridia

SSRI, dopamine and norepinephrine reuptake inhibitor; antiobesity drug
PRC: C; CSS: IV

Available forms
Capsules: 5, 10, 15 mg

Indications & dosages
➤ *Obesity*—**Adult:** 10 mg PO daily. Increase to 15 mg daily after 4 wk prn. Reduce to 5 mg daily if 10-mg dose not tolerated. Max, 15 mg/d.

sildenafil citrate
Viagra

Selective cGMP-specific PDE5 inhibitor; erectile dysfunction drug
PRC: B

Available forms
Tablets: 25, 50, 100 mg

Indications & dosages
➤ *Erectile dysfunction*—**Adult < 65 yr:** 50 mg PO prn 1 hr before sexual activity. Range, 25-100 mg. Max, 1 dose daily. **Elderly:** 25 mg PO prn 1 hr before sexual activity. Adjust prn. Max 1 dose daily.†, ‡

simvastatin
Zocor

HMG-CoA reductase inhibitor; antilipemic
PRC: X

Available forms
Tablets: 5, 10, 20, 40, 80 mg

Indications & dosages
➤ *To prevent CAD; hyperlipidemia*—**Adult:** 20-40 mg PO daily in pm. Adjust dose at intervals ≥ 4 wk prn; range, 5-80 mg/d.†

➤ *Homozygous familial hypercholesterolemia*—**Adult:** 40 mg PO daily in pm or 80 mg PO daily in 3 divided doses (20, 20, and 40 mg in pm).†

➤ *Heterozygous familial hypercholesterolemia*—**Child 10-17 yr:** 10 mg PO q pm. Max 40 mg/d. †

➤ *To reduce risk of CAD mortality and CV events in patients at high risk of coronary events*—**Adult:** 20 mg PO daily in pm. Adjust dosage q 4 wk based on patient tolerance and response. Max, 80 mg daily. **Patient using cyclosporine:** 5 mg PO daily; max, 10 mg/d. **Patient using fibrates or niacin:** Max, 10 mg daily. **Patient using amiodarone or verapamil:** Max, 20 mg daily.

sodium bicarbonate
Bell/ans, Citrocarbonate, Soda Mint

Alkalinizer; systemic and urinary alkalinizer
PRC: C

Available forms
Tablets: 325, 650 mg; *Injection:* 4% (2.4 mEq/5 ml), 4.2% (5 mEq/10 ml), 5% (297.5 mEq/500 ml), 7.5% (8.92 mEq/10 ml and 44.6 mEq/50 ml), 8.4% (10 mEq/10 ml and 50 mEq/50 ml)

Indications & dosages
➤ *Cardiac arrest*—**Adult:** Not routinely recommended; 300-500 ml 5% solution or 200-300 mEq 7.5% or 8.4% solution rapid IV. Base further doses on subsequent blood gas values. Or, 1 mEq/kg dose; repeat 0.5 mEq/kg q 10 min. **Child ≤ 2 yr:** 1 mEq/kg IV or intraosseous injec-

tion of 4.2%-8.4% solution. Give slowly. Max, 8 mEq/kg/d.

➤ *Severe metabolic acidosis*—**Adult:** Dose depends on CO_2, pH, and clinical condition. Generally, 90-180 mEq/L IV during 1st hr; adjust prn.

➤ *Metabolic acidosis*—**Adult, child ≥ 12 yr:** 2-5 mEq/kg as 4-8 hr IV infusion.

➤ *Urinary alkalization*—**Adult:** 48 mEq (4 g) PO, then 12-24 mEq (1-2 g) q 4 hr. May need doses of 30-48 mEq (2.5-4 g) q 4 hr, up to 192 mEq (16 g)/d. **Child:** 1-10 mEq (84-840 mg)/kg PO daily.

➤ *Antacid*—**Adult:** 300 mg-2 g PO daily to qid.

sodium polystyrene sulfonate
Kayexalate, SPS

Cation-exchange resin; potassium-removing resin
PRC: C

Available forms
Powder: 1-pound jar (3.5 g/tsp); *Suspension:* 15 g/60 ml

Indications & dosages
➤ *Hyperkalemia*—**Adult:** 15 g PO daily to qid in H_2O or sorbitol (3-4 ml/g resin). Or, mix powder and give via NG tube. Or, 30-50 g/100 ml sorbitol q 6 hr as warm emulsion 20 cm into sigmoid colon. **Child:** 1 g/kg/dose PO or PR prn. PO route preferred.

sotalol
Betapace, Betapace AF, Sotacor*

Beta blocker; antiarrhythmic
PRC: B

Available forms
Tablets (Betapace): 80, 120, 160, 240 mg; *Tablets (Betapace AF):* 80, 120, 160 mg

Indications & dosages
➤ *Ventricular arrhythmias*—**Adult:** 80 mg PO bid. Increase q 2-3 d prn; range, 160-320 mg/d. †

➤ *Maintain normal sinus rhythm in symptomatic atrial fibrillation or flutter*—**Adult:** 80 mg Betapace AF PO bid. Increase prn to 120 mg PO bid after 3 d if QTc interval < 500 milliseconds. If QTc ≥ 500 milliseconds, reduce dose or stop drug. Max, 160 mg bid.†

spironolactone
Aldactone, Novo-Spiroton*

Potassium-sparing diuretic; anti-hypertensive, diuretic
PRC: NR

Available forms
Tablets: 25, 50, 100 mg

Indications & dosages
➤ *Edema*—**Adult:** 25-200 mg PO daily or in divided doses. **Child:** 3.3 mg/kg PO daily or in divided doses.

➤ *HTN*—**Adult:** 50-100 mg PO daily or in divided doses.

➤ *Diuretic-induced hypokalemia*—**Adult:** 25-100 mg PO daily.

---

streptokinase
Streptase

Plasminogen activator; thrombolytic enzyme
PRC: C

Available forms
Injection: 250,000, 750,000, 1.5 million units in vials for reconstitution

Indications & dosages
➤ *Atrioveous cannula occlusion*—**Adult:** 250,000 units in 2 ml IV solution in each cannula limb over 25-35 min. Clamp cannula × 2 hr. Aspirate, flush, and reconnect.
➤ *Venous thrombosis, PE, arterial thrombosis and embolism*—**Adult:** 250,000 units IV over 30 min. Then 100,000 units/hr IV × 72 hr for DVT and 100,000 units/hr × 24-72 hr for PE and arterial thrombosis or embolism.
➤ *Lysis of coronary artery thrombi*—**Adult:** 20,000 units bolus via coronary catheter; then 2,000 units/min infusion over 60 min. Max dose, 140,000 units. Or, as IV infusion. Usual adult dose 1.5 million units IV over 60 min.

sucralfate
Carafate, Sulcrate*

Pepsin inhibitor; antiulcerative
PRC: B

Available forms
Suspension: 1 g/10 ml; *Tablets:* 1 g

Indications & dosages
➤ *Duodenal ulcer*—**Adult:** 1 g PO qid 1 hr pc and hs × 4-8 wk. May stop therapy sooner if healing shown on endoscopic or radiographic exam.
➤ *Maintenance treatment of duodenal ulcer*—**Adult:** 1 g PO bid.

sulfasalazine (salazosulfapyridine, sulphasalazine)
Azulfidine, Azulfidine EN-tabs

Sulfonamide; antibiotic
PRC: B

Available forms
Tablets: 500 mg; *Tablets (delayed-release):* 500 mg

Indications & dosages
➤ *Ulcerative colitis, Crohn's disease*—**Adult:** 3-4 g/d PO in evenly divided doses; maintenance, 2 g/d PO in divided doses q 6 hr. **Child > 2 yr:** 40-60 mg/kg/d PO, divided into 3-6 doses; then 30 mg/kg/d in 4 doses.
➤ *RA*—**Adult:** 2-3 g/d PO in 2 divided doses.
➤ *Juvenile RA*—**Child ≥ 6 yr:** 30-50 mg/kg delayed-release tablets PO daily in 2 divided doses. Max, 2 g/d. To reduce GI upset, start with ¼-⅓ of maintenance dose and increase q wk × 1 mo.

---

§ Adjust in immunocompromised patients   ¶ Adjust in debilitated patients

sulindac
Apo-Sulin*, Clinoril, Novo-Sundac*

NSAID; nonopioid analgesic, anti-inflammatory
PRC: NR

Available forms
Tablets: 150, 200 mg

Indications & dosages
➤ *OA, RA, ankylosing spondylitis*—**Adult:** 150 mg PO bid; increase to 200 mg bid prn.
➤ *Subacromial bursitis, supraspinatus tendinitis, gouty arthritis*—**Adult:** 200 mg PO bid × 7-14 d. Reduce as symptoms subside.

sumatriptan succinate
Imitrex, Imitrex Nasal Spray

Selective 5-hydroxytryptamine receptor agonist; antimigraine drug
PRC: C

Available forms
Injection: 6 mg/0.5 ml in 0.5-ml prefilled syringes, vials; *Spray:* 5, 20 mg/0.1 ml; *Tablets:* 25, 50, 100 mg (base)

Indications & dosages
➤ *Migraine*—**Adult:** 6 mg SC. Max two 6-mg injections daily ≥ 1 hr apart. Or, initial dose, 25-100 mg PO; 2nd dose, ≤ 100 mg in 2 hr prn. Then, more doses q 2 hr prn; max PO dose, 300 mg/d. Or, 5, 10, or 20 mg intranasally into 1 nostril. May repeat once after 2 hr; max, 40 mg/d.‡

tacrine hydrochloride
Cognex

Cholinesterase inhibitor; psychotherapeutic
PRC: C

Available forms
Capsules: 10, 20, 30, 40 mg

Indications & dosages
➤ *Alzheimer's dementia*—**Adult:** 10 mg PO qid. After 4 wk (if tolerated with no increase in transaminase level), 20 mg qid. After 4 wk, 30 mg qid. If still tolerated, 40 mg qid after another 4 wk. Max, 40 mg qid.

tacrolimus
Protopic

Macrolide; immunosuppressant
PRC: C

Available forms
Ointment: 0.03, 0.1%

Indications & dosages
➤ *Moderate to severe atopic dermatitis where other therapy is inadequate or contraindicated*—**Adult:** Thin layer of 0.03% or 0.1% ointment to affected area bid × 1 wk after area clears. **Child ≥ 2 yr:** Thin layer of 0.03% ointment to affected area bid × 1 wk after area clears.

---

tadalafil
Cialis

Selective cGMP-specific PDE5 inhibitor; erectile dysfunction drug
PRC: B

Available forms
Tablets (film-coated): 5, 10, 20 mg

Indications & dosages
➤ *Erectile dysfunction*—**Man:** 10 mg PO prn before sexual activity. Range 5-20 mg based on effectiveness and tolerance. Max, 1 dose daily. †, ‡ **Patients taking potent CYP 3A4 inhibitors (such as erythromycin, itraconazole, ketoconazole, or ritonavir):** Max, 10 mg q 72 hr.

tamoxifen citrate
Nolvadex, Nolvadex-D*

Nonsteroidal antiestrogen; antineoplastic
PRC: D

Available forms
Tablets: 10, 20 mg; *Tablets (enteric-coated)* *:* 10, 20 mg

Indications & dosages
➤ *Breast CA*—**Adult:** 20-40 mg PO daily. Give doses > 20 mg in 2 divided doses.
➤ *Ductal carcinoma in situ; to reduce risk of invasive breast CA after breast surgery and radiation; to reduce risk of breast CA in high-risk women*—**Adult:** 20 mg PO daily × 5 yr.

tamsulosin hydrochloride
Flomax

Alpha$_{1a}$-antagonist; BPH drug
PRC: B

Available forms
Capsule: 0.4 mg

Indications & dosages
➤ *BPH*—**Man:** 0.4 mg PO daily. If no response after 2-4 wk, increase to 0.8 mg PO daily. If therapy interrupted × several d, restart at 1 capsule daily.

tegaserod maleate
Zelnorm

5-HT$_4$ receptor partial agonist; irritable bowel drug
PRC: B

Available forms
Tablets: 2, 6 mg

Indications & dosages
➤ *IBS with constipation*—**Woman:** 6 mg PO bid ac × 4-6 wk. May repeat × 4-6 wk.

temazepam
Restoril

Benzodiazepine; sedative-hypnotic
PRC: X; CSS: IV

Available forms
Capsules: 15, 30 mg

---

§ Adjust in immunocompromised patients　　　　¶ Adjust in debilitated patients

Indications & dosages
➤ *Insomnia*—**Adult:** 7.5-30 mg PO hs. ¶
Elderly: 7.5 mg PO hs.

tenecteplase
TNKase

Recombinant tissue plasminogen activator; thrombolytic
PRC: C

Available forms
Injection: 50 mg

Indications & dosages
➤ *MI*—**Adult < 60 kg:** 30 mg IV over 5 sec. **Adult 60-69 kg:** 35 mg IV over 5 sec. **Adult 70-79 kg:** 40 mg IV over 5 sec. **Adult 80-89 kg:** 45 mg IV over 5 sec. **Adult ≥ 90 kg:** 50 mg IV over 5 sec. Max 50 mg.

tenofovir disoproxil fumarate
Viread

Nucleotide reverse transcriptase inhibitor; antiviral, antiretroviral
PRC: B

Available forms
Tablets: 300 mg as the fumarate salt (equivalent to 245 mg of tenofovir disoproxil)

Indications & dosages
➤ *HIV-1 infection, with other antiretrovirals*—**Adult:** 300 mg PO daily with meal. Give 2 hr before or 1 hr after didanosine.

terazosin hydrochloride
Hytrin

Selective alpha₁ blocker; antihypertensive
PRC: C

Available forms
Tablets, capsules: 1, 2, 5, 10 mg

Indications & dosages
➤ *HTN*—**Adult:** 1 mg PO hs. Adjust prn. Range 1-5 mg/d; max 20 mg/d.
➤ *Symptomatic BPH*—**Man:** 1 mg PO hs. Increase stepwise to 2, 5, or 10 mg/d; usually 10 mg/d.

terbinafine hydrochloride (oral)
Lamisil

Synthetic allylamine derivative; antifungal
PRC: B

Available forms
Tablets: 250 mg

Indications & dosages
➤ *Tinea unguium*—**Adult:** 250 mg PO daily × 6 wk (fingernail) or × 12 wk (toenail).

terbutaline sulfate
Brethine, Bricanyl

Beta₂ adrenergic agonist; bronchodilator, premature labor inhibitor (tocolytic)
PRC: B

Available forms
Injection: 1 mg/ml; *Tablets:* 2.5, 5 mg

Indications & dosages
➤ *Bronchospasm*—**Adult, child ≥ 12 yr:** 0.25 mg SC; repeat in 15-30 min prn. Max 0.5 mg in 4 hr. Or, 2.5-5 mg PO q 6 hr tid. Max, 15 mg/d. **Child 12-15 yr:** 2.5 mg PO q 6 hr tid while awake. Max, 7.5 mg/d.

teriparatide
Forteo

Biosynthetic parathyroid hormone; antiosteoporotic
PRC: C

Available forms
Injection: 250 mcg/ml

Indications & dosages
➤ *Osteoporosis in high-risk postmenopausal woman or in high-risk man*—**Adult:** 20 mcg SC daily.

testosterone
Testamone 100

testosterone cypionate
Depo-Testosterone

testosterone propionate
Testex

testosterone transdermal system
Androderm, Testoderm

Androgen; androgen replacement, antineoplastic
PRC: X; CSS: III

Available forms
testosterone *Injection (aqueous suspension):* 25, 50, 100 mg/ml; **cypionate** *Injection (in oil):* 100, 200 mg/ml; **propionate** *Injection (in oil):* 50, 100 mg/ml; **transdermal system** *Transdermal patch:* 2.5, 4, 5, 6 mg/d

Indications & dosages
➤ *Hypogonadism*—**Man:** 10-25 mg propionate IM 2-3 times/wk; or 50-400 mg cypionate IM q 2-4 wk.
➤ *Breast CA 1-5 yr postmenopausal*—**Woman:** 100 mg IM twice/wk; 50-100 mg propionate IM 3 times/wk; or 200-400 mg cypionate IM q 2-4 wk.
➤ *Primary, hypogonadotropic hypogonadism*—**Man:** One 4-6 mg/d Testoderm patch on scrotal area daily. Patch worn × 22-24 hr/d; or, two Androderm systems applied pm. Apply to clean, dry skin on back, abdomen, upper arms, or thigh.

tetracycline hydrochloride
Achromycin, Apo-Tetra*, Novo-Tetra*, Nu-Tetra*, Sumycin, Topicycline*

Tetracycline; antibiotic
PRC: D

Available forms
Capsules: 250, 500 mg; *Ointment:* 3%; *Oral suspension:* 125 mg/5 ml; *Topical solution:* 2.2 mg/ml

Indications & dosages
➤ *Infection*—**Adult:** 250-500 mg PO q 6 hr. **Child > 8 yr:** 25-50 mg/kg/d PO in divided doses q 6 hr.

---

§ Adjust in immunocompromised patients   ¶ Adjust in debilitated patients

➤ Chlamydia trachomatis *infection*—
Adult: 500 mg PO qid × 7 d.
➤ *Brucellosis*—**Adult:** 500 mg PO q 6 hr × 3 wk with streptomycin IM.

theophylline
Immediate-release: Bronkodyl,
Slo-Phyllin; timed-release: Aerolate,
Theochron, Theolair, Theo-Sav, T-Phyl,
Uniphyl

theophylline sodium glycinate

Xanthine derivative; bronchodilator
PRC: C

Available forms
Capsules: 100, 200 mg; *Capsules (extended-release):* 50, 60, 75, 100, 125, 130, 200, 250, 260, 300 mg; *D₅W injection:* 200 mg in 50, 100 ml; 400 mg in 100, 250, 500, 1,000 ml; 800 mg in 250, 500, 1,000 ml; *Elixir, oral solution, syrup:* 27, 50 mg/5 ml; *Tablets:* 100, 125, 200, 250, 300 mg; *Tablets (chewable):* 100 mg; *Tablets (extended-release):* 100, 200, 250, 300, 400, 500, 600 mg

Indications & dosages
➤ *Acute bronchospasm if not already using drug*—IV loading dose, 4.7 mg/kg slowly; then maintenance. **Adult nonsmoker:** 6 mg/kg PO; then 2-3 mg/kg q 6 hr × 2 doses. Maintenance, 3 mg/kg q 8 hr. Or, 0.55 mg/kg/hr IV × 12 hr; then 0.39 mg/kg/hr. **Healthy adult smoker, child 9-16 yr:** 6 mg/kg PO; then 3 mg/kg q 4 hr × 3 doses. Maintenance, 3 mg/kg q 6 hr. Or, 0.79 mg/kg/hr IV × 12 hr; then

0.63 mg/kg/hr. **Adult with HF, liver disease:** 6 mg/kg PO; then 2 mg/kg q 8 hr × 2 doses. Maintenance 1-2 mg/kg q 12 hr. Or, 0.39 mg/kg/hr IV × 12 hr; then 0.08-0.16 mg/kg/hr. **Child 6 mo-9 yr:** 6 mg/kg PO; then 4 mg/kg q 4 hr × 3 doses. Maintenance, 4 mg/kg q 6 hr. Or, 0.95 mg/kg/hr IV × 12 hr; then 0.79 mg/kg/hr.
➤ *Chronic bronchospasm*—**Adult, child:** 16 mg/kg or 400 mg PO daily in 3-4 divided doses q 6-8 hr; or 12 mg/kg or 400 mg (extended-release) PO daily in 2 or 3 divided doses q 8 or 12 hr. Increase as tolerated q 2 or 3 d to max. **Child > 16 yr:** 13 mg/kg or 900 mg PO daily in divided doses. **Child 12-16 yr:** 18 mg/kg PO daily in divided doses. **Child 9-12 yr:** 20 mg/kg PO daily in divided doses. **Child < 9 yr:** 24 mg/kg/d PO in divided doses.

thiamine hydrochloride (vitamin B₁)
Biamine

Water-soluble vitamin; nutritional supplement
PRC: A

Available forms
Elixir*: 250 mcg/5 ml; *Injection:* 100 mg/ml; *Tablets:* 25, 50, 100, 250, 500 mg; *Tablets (enteric-coated):* 20 mg

Indications & dosages
➤ *Beriberi*—**Adult:** 10-20 mg IM tid × 2 wk; then diet correction and multivitamin containing 5-10 mg/d thiamine × 1 mo. **Child:** 10-50 mg/d IM × several wk with adequate diet.

➤ *Wernicke's encephalopathy*—**Adult:** 100 mg IV; then 50-100 mg/d IV or IM until patient eats balanced diet.

thioridazine hydrochloride
Apo-Thioridazine*, Mellaril, Mellaril Concentrate, Novo-Ridazine*, PMS Thioridazine*

Phenothiazine (piperidine derivative); antipsychotic
PRC: NR

Available forms
Oral concentrate: 30, 100 mg/ml (3-4.2% alcohol); *Oral suspension:* 25, 100 mg/5 ml; *Tablets:* 10, 15, 25, 50, 100, 150, 200 mg

Indications & dosages
➤ *Psychosis not responsive to other drugs*—**Adult:** 50-100 mg PO tid; slowly increase to 800 mg/d in divided doses prn. **Child:** Initially, 0.5 mg/kg/d PO in divided doses. May increase gradually to max of 3 mg/kg/d.

thiothixene

thiothixene hydrochloride
Navane

Thioxanthene; antipsychotic
PRC: NR

Available forms
thiothixene *Capsules:* 1, 2, 5, 10, 20 mg; **hydrochloride** *Oral concentrate:* 5 mg/ml (7% alcohol)

Indications & dosages
➤ *Psychosis*—**Adult:** 2 mg PO tid. Increase to 15 mg/d.
➤ *Severe psychosis*—**Adult:** 5 mg PO bid. Increase to 20-30 mg/d. Max 60 mg/d.

ticarcillin disodium
Ticar

Extended-spectrum PCN, alpha-carboxypenicillin; antibiotic
PRC: B

Available forms
Powder for injection: 1, 3, 6 g; *IV infusion:* 3 g

Indications & dosages
➤ *Serious infection*—**Adult:** 200-300 mg/kg IV daily in divided doses q 4-6 hr.†,‡ **Child < 40 kg:** 200-300 mg/kg IV daily in divided doses q 4-6 hr.†, ‡ **Neonate > 2 kg:** 225-300 mg/kg daily in divided doses q 8 hr IM or IV over 10-20 min.†,‡ **Neonate < 2 kg:** 150-225 mg/kg daily in divided doses q 8-12 hr IM or IV over 10-20 min.†, ‡
➤ *UTI*—**Adult, child:** Complicated infection, 150-200 mg/kg IV daily in divided doses q 4-6 hr. **Adult:** Uncomplicated infection, 1 g IV or IM q 6 hr.†, ‡ **Child < 40 kg:** Uncomplicated infection, 50-100 mg/kg daily IM or direct IV divided q 6-8 hr.†, ‡

ticarcillin disodium and clavulanate potassium
Timentin

Beta-lactamase inhibitor; antibiotic
PRC: B

Available forms
Injection: 3 g ticarcillin and 100 mg clavulanic acid

Indications & dosages
➤ *UTI; lower respiratory tract, bone and joint, skin and skin-structure infection; septicemia*—**Adult:** 3.1 g IV infusion q 4-6 hr.†

ticlopidine hydrochloride
Ticlid

Platelet aggregation inhibitor; antithrombotic
PRC: B

Available forms
Tablets: 250 mg

Indications & dosages
➤ *Reduce risk of thrombotic stroke*—**Adult:** 250 mg PO bid with meals.

timolol maleate (ophthalmic)
Betimol, Timoptic, Timoptic-XE

Beta blocker; antiglaucoma drug
PRC: C

Available forms
Ophthalmic solution, gel: 0.25, 0.5%

Indications & dosages
➤ *Chronic glaucoma, elevated IOP from ocular HTN*—**Adult:** 1 drop 0.25% solution in each affected eye bid; maintenance 1 drop/d. If no response, 1 drop 0.5% solution bid. If IOP is controlled, reduce to 1 drop/d. Or, 1 drop gel daily.

timolol maleate (systemic)
Apo-Timol*, Blocadren

Beta blocker; antihypertensive, adjunct in MI treatment
PRC: C

Available forms
Tablets: 5, 10, 20 mg

Indications & dosages
➤ *HTN*—**Adult:** 10 mg PO bid. Max, 60 mg/d. Increase q wk prn.
➤ *MI*—**Adult:** 10 mg PO bid.
➤ *To prevent migraine*—**Adult:** 20 mg PO daily in 1 or divided doses bid. Increase prn to max 30 mg/d.

tinzaparin sodium
Innohep

Low–molecular-weight heparin; anticoagulant
PRC: B

Available forms
Injection: 20,000 anti-Xa IU per ml in 2-ml vials

---

*Canadian   † Adjust in renal impairment   ‡ Adjust in liver impairment

Indications & dosages
➤ *Symptomatic DVT with or without PE*—**Adult:** 175 anti-Xa IU/kg SC daily × ≥ 6 d and until patient is adequately anticoagulated with warfarin (INR ≥ 2.0) × 2 consecutive d. Warfarin treatment should begin when appropriate, usually within 1-3 d after drug starts. Volume to be given may be calculated as follows: Patient wt in kg × 0.00875 ml/kg = volume to be given (in ml).

tobramycin
AKTob, Tobrex

Aminoglycoside; antibiotic
PRC: B

Available forms
Ophthalmic ointment, solution: 0.3%

Indications & dosages
➤ *Ocular infection*—**Adult, child:** 1 or 2 drops into affected eye q 4 hr, or thin strip (1 cm) ointment q 8-12 hr. In severe infection, 2 drops into infected eye q 30-60 min until improvement; then reduce frequency. Or, thin strip ointment q 3-4 hr until improvement; then reduce frequency.

tobramycin sulfate
Nebcin, TOBI

Aminoglycoside; antibiotic
PRC: D

Available forms
Injection: 80, 20 (pediatric) mg/2 ml; *Nebulizer solution (for inhalation):*

300 mg/5 ml; *Premixed parenteral injection for IV infusion:* 60, 80 mg in NSS

Indications & dosages
➤ *Serious infection*—**Adult:** 3 mg/kg/d IM or IV divided q 8 hr. Max, 5 mg/kg/d divided q 6-8 hr for life-threatening infection; reduce to 3 mg/kg/d as soon as indicated. **Child:** 6-7.5 mg/kg/d IM or IV in 3 or 4 equally divided doses. **Neonate < 1 wk, premature infant:** Up to 4 mg/kg/d IV or IM in 2 equal doses q 12 hr.†
➤ *Pseudomonas aeruginosa infection in cystic fibrosis*—**Adult, child ≥ 6 yr:** 300 mg q 12 hr via nebulizer × 28 d, followed by 28 d without drug. Repeat cycle.

tolcapone
Tasmar

Catechol-O-methyltransferase inhibitor; antiparkinsonian
PRC: C

Available forms
Tablets: 100, 200 mg

Indications & dosages
➤ *Parkinson's disease*—**Adult:** 100 mg PO tid (with levodopa and carbidopa). Recommended daily dose, 100 mg PO tid; 200 mg PO tid can be given, if needed. If giving 200 mg tid and dyskinesia occurs, may reduce levodopa. Max, 600 mg/d.

---

§ Adjust in immunocompromised patients   ¶ Adjust in debilitated patients

tolterodine tartrate
Detrol, Detrol LA

Muscarinic receptor antagonist; anticholinergic
PRC: C

Available forms
Capsules (extended-release): 2, 4 mg;
Tablets: 1, 2 mg

Indications & dosages
➤ *Overactive bladder*—**Adult:** 2 mg PO
bid. May lower to 1 mg bid, based on response and tolerance. Or, 4 mg extended-release PO daily. May reduce to 2 mg
extended-release daily.‡

topiramate
Topamax

*Sulfamate-substituted monosaccharide;
antiepileptic*
PRC: C

Available forms
Sprinkle capsules: 15, 25 mg; *Tablets:* 25,
100, 200 mg

Indications & dosages
➤ *Partial-onset seizures; primary generalized tonic-clonic seizures*—**Adult:** Start
doses at 25-50 mg/d PO, then adjust to
25-50 mg/wk. Adjust to dosing of 200-
400 mg/d in 2 divided doses for partial
seizures and 400 mg/d in 2 divided doses
for generalized tonic-clonic.†
➤ *Partial seizures, primary generalized
tonic-clonic seizures, or Lennox-Gastaut
syndrome*—**Child 2-16 yr:** 5-9 mg/kg/d
PO in 2 divided doses. Begin dosage adjustment at 1-3 mg/kg pm × 1 wk. Increase at 1-2 wk intervals by 1-3 mg/kg/d
to achieve optimum response. Adjust
dose according to response.†

tramadol hydrochloride
Ultram

Synthetic analgesic; analgesic
PRC: C

Available forms
Tablets: 50 mg

Indications & dosages
➤ *Pain*—**Adult < 75 yr:** 50-100 mg PO
q 4-6 hr prn. Max, 400 mg/d. **Elderly
> 75 yr:** Max, 300 mg/d in divided
doses.†, ‡

trazodone hydrochloride
Desyrel

Triazolopyridine derivative; antidepressant
PRC: C

Available forms
Tablets: 50, 100, 150, 300 mg

Indications & dosages
➤ *Depression*—**Adult:** 150 mg PO daily
in divided doses; increase by 50 mg/d q
3-4 d prn. Average dosage, 150-
400 mg/d. Max dosage, 600 mg/d
(inpatient); 400 mg/d (outpatient).

---

*Canadian   † Adjust in renal impairment   ‡ Adjust in liver impairment

treprostinil sodium
Remodulin

Vasodilator; antihypertensive
PRC: B

Available forms
Injection: 1 mg/ml, 2.5 mg/ml, 5 mg/ml, 10 mg/ml

Indications & dosages
➤ *To reduce symptoms of New York Heart Association class II to IV pulmonary arterial hypertension caused by exercise*—**Adult:** 1.25 ng/kg/min continuous SC infusion. May reduce initial dose to 0.625 ng/kg/min prn. Increase by ≤ 1.25 ng/kg/min q wk for the 1st 4 wk and then by ≤ 2.5 ng/kg/min each wk for remaining duration of treatment. Don't stop abruptly. Max, 40 ng/kg/min.‡

tretinoin (retinoic acid, vitamin A acid)
Avita, Renova, Retin-A, Retin-A Micro, Stieva-A*, Stieva-A Forte*

Retinoid, vitamin A derivative; anti-acne agent, anti-wrinkle agent
PRC: C

Available forms
Cream: 0.02, 0.025, 0.05, 0.1%; *Gel:* 0.01, 0.025%; *Microsphere gel:* 0.04%, 0.1%; *Solution:* 0.05%

Indications & dosages
➤ *Acne*—**Adult, child:** Clean affected area and lightly apply daily hs.

➤ *Fine facial wrinkles*—**Adult:** Apply small, pearl-sized amount 0.02% cream to cover area lightly, q pm. May increase to 0.05% cream if skin care and sun-avoidance program alone don't work.

triamcinolone acetonide (systemic)
Azmacort, Kenalog-10, Triamonide 40, Trilog

Glucocorticoid; anti-inflammatory, anti-asthmatic
PRC: C

Available forms
Inhalation aerosol: 100 mcg/metered spray; *Injection (suspension):* 3, 10, 40 mg/ml; *Tablets:* 4 mg

Indications & dosages
➤ *Inflammation, immunosuppression*—**Adult:** 4-48 mg/d PO in divided doses; 40 mg IM wkly; 1 mg into lesions; 2.5-40 mg into joints or soft tissue.
➤ *Asthma*—**Adult:** 2 inhalations Azmacort tid or qid, or 4 inhalations given bid. Max, 16 inhalations/d. **Child 6-12 yr:** 1 or 2 inhalations Azmacort tid or qid, or 2-4 inhalations given bid. Max, 12 inhalations/d.

trifluoperazine hydrochloride

Apo-Trifluoperazine*, Solazine*, Terfluzine*

Phenothiazine (piperazine derivative); antipsychotic
PRC: NR

Available forms

Injection: 2 mg/ml; *Oral concentration:* 10 mg/ml; *Tablets:* 1, 2, 5, 10 mg

Indications & dosages

➤ *Anxiety*—**Adult:** 1-2 mg PO bid. Max, 6 mg/d. Don't give > 12 wk.
➤ *Schizophrenia, other psychotic disorders*—**Hospitalized or closely supervised adult:** 2-5 mg PO bid, increase until response. Or, 1-2 mg deep IM q 4-6 hr prn; > 6 mg IM/24 hr rarely needed. **Hospitalized or closely supervised child 6-12 yr:** 1 mg PO daily or bid; may increase to 15 mg/d. Or, 1 mg IM up to bid at least 4 hr apart.

trihexyphenidyl hydrochloride

Apo-Trihex*, Trihexy-2, Trihexy-5

Anticholinergic; antiparkinsonian
PRC: NR

Available forms

Tablets: 2, 5 mg

Indications & dosages

➤ *Parkinsonism*—**Adult:** 1 mg PO d 1, 2 mg d 2; then increase by 2 mg q 3-5 d until total of 6-10 mg/d. Give tid with

meals or qid or as extended-release form bid. In post-encephalitic parkinsonism, 12-15 mg/d may be needed.

triptorelin pamoate

Trelstar Depot, Trelstar LA

Synthetic luteinizing hormone-releasing hormone analogue; antineoplastic
PRC: X

Available forms

Injection: 3.75-, 11.25-mg single-dose vials and Debioclip single-dose delivery system

Indications & dosages

➤ *Palliative therapy for advanced prostate CA*—**Man:** 3.75 mg IM Trelstar Depot q mo as single injection or 11.25 mg IM Trelstar LA given q 84 d as single injection.

valacyclovir hydrochloride

Valtrex

Synthetic purine nucleoside; antiviral
PRC: B

Available forms

Caplets: 500, 1,000 mg

Indications & dosages

➤ *Herpes zoster (shingles)*—**Adult:** 1 g PO tid × 7 d.†
➤ *Initial genital herpes*—**Adult:** 1 g PO bid × 10 d.†
➤ *Recurrent genital herpes*—**Adult:** 500 mg PO bid × 3 d at 1st sign.†,§

---

*Canadian   † Adjust in renal impairment   ‡ Adjust in liver impairment

➤ *Chronic suppression of recurrent genital herpes*—**Adult:** 1 g PO daily. Patient with ≤ 9 episodes/yr can take 500 mg PO daily.†.§
➤ *To reduce risk of transmitting genital herpes in patients with a history of ≤ 9 recurrences/yr*—**Adult:** 500 mg PO daily.†
➤ *Cold sores (herpes labialis)*—**Adult:** 2g PO × 2 doses, about 12 hr apart.†

valdecoxib
Bextra

COX-2 inhibitor; NSAID
PRC: C

Available forms
Tablets: 10, 20 mg

Indications & dosages
➤ *OA, RA*—**Adult:** 10 mg PO daily.
➤ *Primary dysmenorrhea*—**Adult:** 20 mg PO bid prn.

valganciclovir
Valcyte

Synthetic nucleoside; antiviral
PRC: C

Available forms
Tablets: 450 mg

Indications & dosages
➤ *Active CMV retinitis in AIDS*—**Adult:** 900 mg PO bid with food × 21 d. Maintenance, 900 mg daily with food.†
➤ *Inactive CMV retinitis*—**Adult:** 900 mg PO daily with food.†

➤ *To prevent CMV disease in heart, kidney, and kidney-pancreas transplantation patients at high risk*—**Adult:** 900 mg PO daily with food starting within 10 d of transplantation until 100 d post-transplantation.†

valproate sodium
Depacon, Depakene Syrup

valproic acid
Depakene

divalproex sodium
Depakote, Depakote ER, Depakote Sprinkle, Epival*

Carboxylic acid derivative; anticonvulsant
PRC: D

Available forms
valproate *Injection:* 100 mg/ml; *Syrup:* 250 mg/5 ml; **valproic** *Capsules:* 250 mg; **divalproex** *Capsules (sprinkle):* 125 mg; *Tablets (delayed-release):* 125, 250, 500 mg; *Tablets (extended-release):* 250, 500 mg

Indications & dosages
➤ *Simple and complex absence seizures, mixed seizure types (including absence seizures)*—**Adult, child:** 15 mg/kg PO or IV daily; increase by 5-10 mg/kg/d q wk to max 60 mg/kg/d. Don't use Depakote ER in child < 10 yr.
➤ *Mania*—**Adult:** 750 mg/d divalproex sodium in divided doses. Adjust prn; max 60 mg/kg/d.

---

§ Adjust in immunocompromised patients　　　　¶ Adjust in debilitated patients

➤ *To prevent migraine*—**Adult:** 250 mg divalproex sodium delayed-release PO bid; increase to 1,000 mg/d prn. Or, 500 mg Depakote ER PO daily × 1 wk, then 1,000 mg PO daily.

➤ *Complex partial seizures*—**Adult, child ≥ 10 yr:** 10-15 mg/kg Depakote or Depakote ER PO or IV daily; increase by 5-10 mg/kg/d q wk to max 60 mg/kg/d. **Elderly:** Start at lower dose and adjust dose more slowly. Regularly monitor fluid and nutritional intake and for dehydration, somnolence, and other adverse reactions.

valsartan
Diovan

Angiotensin II antagonist; antihypertensive
PRC: C (D, 2nd and 3rd trimesters)

Available forms
Tablets: 40, 80, 160, 320 mg

Indications & dosages
➤ *HTN*—**Adult:** 80 mg PO daily. BP reduction in 2-4 wk. For greater effect, increase to 160 or 320 mg/d or add diuretic.
➤ *HF (New York Heart Association class II-IV) in patients intolerant of ACE inhibitors*—**Adult:** 40 mg PO bid. Increase as tolerated to 80 mg bid. Max, 160 mg bid. Consider reduction in diuretic use. Use with an ACE inhibitor and a beta blocker isn't recommended.

vancomycin hydrochloride
Lyphocin, Vancocin, Vancoled

Glycopeptide; antibiotic
PRC: C

Available forms
Capsules: 125, 250 mg; *IV infusion (frozen):* 500 mg/100 ml D₅W; *Powder for injection:* 500-mg, 1-g vial; *Powder for oral solution:* 1-, 10-g bottle

Indications & dosages
➤ *Serious infection*—**Adult:** 1-1.5 g IV q 12 hr. **Child:** 10 mg/kg IV q 6 hr. **Neonate, infant:** 15 mg/kg IV; then 10 mg/kg IV q 12 hr if < 1 wk of age, and 10 mg/kg IV q 8 hr if > 1 wk of age but < 1 mo of age.†
➤ *Pseudomembranous and staphylococcal enterocolitis from antibiotics*—**Adult:** 125-500 mg PO q 6 h × 7-10 d. **Child:** 40 mg/kg PO daily in divided doses q 6 hr × 7-10 d. Max, 2 g/d.†
➤ *Endocarditis prophylaxis (dental procedures)*—**Adult, child > 27 kg:** 1 g IV over 1 hr starting 1 hr before procedure. **Child < 27 kg:** 20 mg/kg IV over 1-2 hr; ending within 30 min of start of procedure.†

vardenafil hydrochloride
Levitra

Selective cGMP-specific PDE5 inhibitor; erectile dysfunction drug
PRC: B

Available forms
Tablets (film-coated): 2.5, 5, 10, 20 mg

Indications & dosages
➤ *Erectile dysfunction*—**Man < 65 yr:** 10 mg PO as a single dose prn 1 hr before sexual activity. Range, 5-20 mg based on effectiveness and tolerance. Max, 1 dose daily. ‡ **Man ≥ 65 yr:** First dose is 5 mg PO daily prn. ‡

venlafaxine hydrochloride
Effexor, Effexor XR

SSRI, norepinephrine, dopamine reuptake inhibitor; antidepressant
PRC: C

Available forms
Capsules (extended-release): 37.5, 75, 150 mg; *Tablets:* 25, 37.5, 50, 75, 100 mg

Indications & dosages
➤ *Depression, anxiety*—**Adult:** 75 mg PO daily in 2 or 3 divided doses with food. For anxiety, use extended-release. Increase prn by 75 mg/d at intervals ≥ 4 d. For moderate depression, max, 225 mg/d. For severe depression, max, 375 mg/d.

verapamil hydrochloride
Apo-Verap*, Calan, Calan SR, Covera-HS, Isoptin SR, Novo-Veramil*, Nu-Verap*, Verelan, Verelan PM

Calcium channel blocker; antianginal, antihypertensive, antiarrhythmic
PRC: C

Available forms
Capsules (extended-release): 120, 180, 240 mg; *Capsules (sustained-release):* 120, 160*, 180, 240, 360 mg; *Injection:* 2.5 mg/ml; *Tablets:* 40, 80, 120 mg; *Tablets (extended-release):* 100, 120, 180, 200, 240, 300 mg; *Tablets (sustained-release):* 120, 180, 240 mg

Indications & dosages
➤ *Vasospastic angina, chronic angina, chronic atrial fibrillation*—**Adult:** 80-120 mg PO tid. Increase q wk prn. Max, 480 mg/d.
➤ *Supraventricular arrhythmias*—**Adult:** 0.075-0.15 mg/kg IV push over 2 min; 0.15 mg/kg in 30 min prn. **Child < 1 yr:** 0.1-0.2 mg/kg IV over 2 min. **Child 1-15 yr:** 0.1-0.3 mg/kg IV over 2 min. For child, may repeat in 30 min.
➤ *HTN*—**Adult:** 120-240 mg PO daily of extended-release capsules or tablets in am; may increase by 120 mg increments. Or, 180 mg Covera-HS PO hs of extended-release core tablets; may increase to 240 mg PO daily; may be further increased by 120 mg increments to max 480 mg. Or, 200 mg (Verelan-PM) controlled extended-release capsule PO daily; may increase to 300-400 mg hs. Or, 40 mg PO immediate-release bid to 80 mg tid; max, 360-480 mg daily.

vinblastine sulfate (VLB)
Velban, Velbe*

Vinca alkaloid; antineoplastic
PRC: D

Available forms
Injection: 10-mg vial (lyophilized powder), 1 mg/ml in 10-ml vials

---

Indications & dosages
➤ *Breast, testicular CA; Hodgkin's disease; malignant lymphoma*—**Adult:** 3.7 mg/m² IV q 1-2 wk. Max, 18.5 mg/m² IV q wk. If WBC < 4,000/mm³, don't repeat. **Child:** 2.5 mg/m² IV q wk. Increase by 1.25 mg/m² until WBC < 3,000/mm³ or tumor responds. Max 12.5 mg/m² IV q wk.‡

vincristine sulfate (VCR)
Oncovin, Vincasar PFS

Vinca alkaloid; antineoplastic
PRC: D

Available forms
Injection: 1 mg/ml in 1-, 2-, 5-ml multidose and preservative-free vials

Indications & dosages
➤ *Acute lymphoblastic leukemia, other leukemias; Hodgkin's disease*—**Adult:** 1.4 mg/m² IV q wk. Max 2 mg/wk. **Child > 10 kg:** 2 mg/m² IV q wk. **Child ≤ 10 kg or body surface area < 1 m²:** Initially, 0.05 mg/kg IV q wk.

voriconazole
Vfend

Synthetic triazole; antifungal
PRC: D

Available forms
Injection: 200 mg; *Tablets:* 50, 200 mg

Indications & dosages
➤ *Invasive aspergillosis; serious infections caused by* Fusarium *species and* Scedosporium apiospermum *in patients intolerant of or refractory to other therapy*—**Adult:** 6 mg/kg IV q 12 hr × 2 doses, then 4 mg/kg IV q 12 hr. Switch to PO form as tolerated, using maintenance doses‡. **Adult ≥ 40 kg:** 200 mg PO q 12 hr. May increase to 300 mg PO q 12 hr prn.‡ **Adult < 40 kg:** 100 mg PO q 12 hr. May increase to 150 mg PO q 12 hr prn.‡
➤ *Esophageal candidiasis*—**Adult ≥ 40 kg:** 200 mg PO q 12 hr. Treat × ≥ 14 d followed by ≥ 7 d after resolution of symptoms. **Adult < 40 kg:** 100 mg PO q 12 hr. Treat × ≥ 14 d followed by ≥ 7 d after resolution of symptoms. ‡

warfarin sodium
Coumadin, Panwarfin, Sofarin, Warfilone

Coumarin derivative; anticoagulant
PRC: X

Available forms
Powder for injection: 2 mg/ml; *Tablets:* 1, 2, 2.5, 3, 4, 5, 6, 7.5, 10 mg

Indications & dosages
➤ *PE with DVT, MI, rheumatic heart disease with heart valve damage, prosthetic heart valves, chronic atrial fibrillation*—**Adult:** 2-5 mg PO daily × 2-4 d; then dose based on daily PT and INR. Maintenance, 2-10 mg PO daily.

zafirlukast
Accolate

Antileukotriene; anti-inflammatory
PRC: B

Available forms

Tablets: 10, 20 mg

Indications & dosages

➤ *Asthma*—**Adult, child ≥ 12 yr:** 20 mg PO bid 1 hr ac or 2 hr pc. **Child 5-11 yr:** 10 mg PO bid.

zalcitabine (ddC, dideoxycytidine)
Hivid

Nucleoside analogue; antiviral
PRC: C

Available forms

Tablets: 0.375, 0.75 mg

Indications & dosages

➤ *Advanced HIV infection*—**Adult, child ≥ 13 yr:** 0.75 mg PO q 8 hr with zidovudine 200 mg PO q 8 hr.†

zaleplon
Sonata

Pyrazolopyrimidine; hypnotic
PRC: C; CSS: IV

Available forms

Capsules: 5, 10 mg

Indications & dosages

➤ *Insomnia (short-term)*—**Adult:** 10 mg PO daily hs; increase to 20 mg prn. Low-wt adult may respond to 5-mg dose.‡,¶

zidovudine (azidothymidine, AZT)
Apo-Zidovudine*, Novo-AZT*, Retrovir

Thymidine analogue; antiviral
PRC: C

Available forms

Capsules: 100 mg; *Injection:* 10 mg/ml; *Syrup:* 50 mg/5 ml; *Tablets:* 300 mg

Indications & dosages

➤ *HIV infection*—**Adult, child ≥ 12 yr:** 600 mg/d PO in divided doses with other antiretrovirals. Or, 1 mg/kg IV over 1 hr q 4 hr until patient can tolerate oral therapy. **Child 6 wk-12 yr:** 160 mg/m^2 PO q 8 hr (480 mg/m^2/d to max 200 mg q 8 hr) or 120 mg/m^2 IV q 6 hr by intermittent infusion or 20 mg/m^2/hr by continuous infusion with other antiretrovirals. †,‡

Hemoglobin < 7.5 g/dl or reduction of > 25% of baseline or granulocyte count < 750 cells/mm^3 or reduction of > 50% from baseline may require interrupting dose until marrow recovery is observed.

➤ *To prevent maternal-fetal HIV transmission*—**Pregnant woman (initiate at 14-34 wk gestation):** 100 mg PO 5 times/d until start of labor. Then, 2 mg/kg IV over 1 hr followed by continuous IV infusion of 1 mg/kg/hr until umbilical cord is clamped. **Neonate:** 2 mg/kg PO q 6 hr starting within 6-12 hr after birth and continuing until 6 wk old. Or, give 1.5 mg/kg IV over 30 min q 6 hr.†, ‡

---

§ Adjust in immunocompromised patients   ¶ Adjust in debilitated patients

ziprasidone
Geodon

Atypical antipsychotic; psychotropic
PRC: C

Available forms
Capsules: 20, 40, 60, 80 mg; *Injection:* 20 mg/ml single-dose vials (after reconstitution)

Indications & dosages
➤ *Symptomatic schizophrenia*—**Adult:** 20 mg PO bid with food. Adjust dosage, if necessary, should occur no sooner than q 2 days, but to ensure lowest possible doses, interval should be several wk to allow symptoms to respond. Effective dosage range, 20-80 mg bid. Max, 100 mg bid.
➤ *Rapid control of acute agitation in schizophrenia*—**Adult:** 10-20 mg IM prn; max 40 mg/d. Doses of 10 mg may be given q 2 hr; doses of 20 mg may be given q 4 hr.

zoledronic acid
Zometa

Bisphosphonate; antihypercalcemic
PRC: D

Available forms
Injection: 4 mg zoledronic acid, 220 mg mannitol, 24 mg sodium citrate

Indications & dosages
➤ *Hypercalcemia from malignancy*— **Adult:** 4 mg IV over ≥ 15 min. If albumin-corrected calcium level doesn't return to normal, may retreat with 4 mg. Allow ≥ 7 d to pass before retreatment to allow full response to initial dose.†
➤ *Multiple myeloma and bone metastases of solid tumors with standard antineoplastic therapy (prostate CA has progressed after at least one hormonal therapy)*—**Adult:** 4 mg IV over 15 min q 3-4 wk.†

zolmitriptan
Zomig, Zomig-ZMT

Selective 5-HT receptor agonist; antimigraine drug
PRC: C

Available forms
Tablets (immediate-release): 2.5, 5 mg; *Tablets (oral disintegrating):* 2.5, 5 mg; *Nasal spray:* 5 mg

Indications & dosages
➤ *Migraine*—**Adult:** 2.5 mg PO; increase to 5 mg/dose prn. Or, 5 mg (1 nasal spray) into nostril. If migraine returns, may give 2nd dose after 2 hr. Max, 10 mg/24 hr.‡

zolpidem tartrate
Ambien

Imidazopyridine; hypnotic
PRC: B; CSS: IV

Available forms
Tablets: 5, 10 mg

Indications & dosages
➤ *Insomnia (short-term)*—**Adult:** 10 mg
PO q hs. **Elderly:** 5 mg PO q hs. Max
10 mg/d.‡

zonisamide
Zonegran

Sulfonamide; anticonvulsant
PRC: C

Available forms
Capsules: 100 mg

Indications & dosages
➤ *Partial seizures*—**Adult, child > 16 yr:**
100 mg PO daily. Increase 100 mg/d q
2 wk prn; max 400 mg/d. For dose >
100 mg, give daily or divide bid.†,‡

Pregnancy Risk Categories

Pregnancy risk categories are assigned by the Food and Drug Administration and reflect a drug's potential to cause birth defects.

- A: Adequate studies in pregnant women haven't shown a risk to the fetus.
- B: Animal studies haven't shown a risk to the fetus, but controlled studies haven't been conducted in pregnant women; or animal studies have shown an adverse effect on the fetus, but adequate studies in pregnant women haven't shown a fetal risk.
- C: Animal studies have shown an adverse effect on the fetus, but adequate studies haven't been conducted in humans. The benefits may be acceptable despite the risks.
- D: The drug may pose a risk to the human fetus, but potential benefits may be worth the risk.
- X: Studies in animals or humans show fetal abnormalities, or reports of adverse reactions indicate evidence of fetal risk. The risks clearly outweigh the potential benefits.
- NR: Not rated.

Controlled Substance Schedules

Drugs regulated under the Controlled Substances Act of 1970 are divided into the following schedules:

- I: High abuse potential, no accepted medical use
- II: High abuse potential, severe dependence danger
- III: Less abuse potential than schedule II drugs, moderate dependence danger
- IV: Less abuse potential than schedule III drugs, limited dependence danger
- V: Limited abuse potential

Dialyzable drugs

The amount of a drug removed by dialysis differs among patients and depends on several factors, including the patient's condition, the drug's properties, the length of dialysis, the dialysate used, the rate of blood flow or dwell time, and the purpose of dialysis. Levels of the following drugs are reduced by dialysis.

acetaminophen (may not influence toxicity)

acyclovir

allopurinol

amikacin

amoxicillin

amoxicillin and clavulanate potassium

ampicillin

ampicillin and sulbactam sodium

aspirin

atenolol

azathioprine

aztreonam

captopril

carbenicillin

cefaclor

cefadroxil

cefazolin

cefepime

cefonicid (by 20%)

cefoperazone

cefotaxime

cefotetan (by 20%)

cefoxitin

cefpodoxime

ceftazidime

ceftibuten

ceftizoxime

cefuroxime

cephalexin

cephalothin

cephradine

chloral hydrate

chloramphenicol (by very small amount)

cimetidine

ciprofloxacin (by 20%)

co-trimoxazole

cyclophosphamide

didanosine

disopyramide

enalapril

erythromycin (by 20%)

ethambutol (by 20%)

famciclovir

fluconazole

flucytosine

fluorouracil

foscarnet

gabapentin

ganciclovir

gentamicin

imipenem and cilastatin
isoniazid
kanamycin
ketoprofen
lisinopril
lithium
loracarbef
mercaptopurine
meropenem
methotrexate
methyldopa
metronidazole
mexiletine
minoxidil
nadolol
nelfinavir
netilmicin
nitrofurantoin
nitroprusside
ofloxacin
penicillin G
pentazocine
perindopril
phenobarbital
piperacillin and tazobactam
primidone
procainamide
pyridoxine
quinidine
ranitidine

sotalol
stavudine
streptomycin
sulbactam
sulfamethoxazole
theophylline
ticarcillin
ticarcillin and clavulanate
tobramycin
tocainide
topiramate
trimethoprim
valacyclovir

Drugs that prolong the QTc interval

Drug-induced prolonged QTc interval most frequently occurs with Class I and III antiarrhythmics, antihistamines, antidepressants, antifungals, and antipsychotics. Grapefruit juice can increase the risk of drug-induced prolonged QTc interval by inhibiting the metabolism of amiodarone.

Patients at high risk include women, children, and patients with hypokalemia, hypomagnesia, renal failure, and heart failure. Selected drugs that may prolong the QTc interval are listed below.

amantadine
amiodarone
aripiprazole
arsenic trioxide
azithromycin
chloral hydrate
chlorpromazine
cisapride
clarithromycin
disopyramide
dofetilide
dolasetron
domperidone
droperidol
erythromycin
felbamate
flecainide
foscarnet
fosphenytoin
gatifloxacin
gemifloxacin
granisetron
halofantrine

haloperidol
ibutilide
indapamide
isradipine
levofloxacin
levomethadyl
lithium
mesoridazine
methadone
moexipril and
hydrochlorothiazide
moxifloxacin
naratriptan
nicardipine
octreotide
ondansetron
pentamidine
pimozide
procainamide
quetiapine
quinidine
risperidone
salmeterol

sotalol
sparfloxacin
sumatriptan
tacrolimus
tamoxifen
thioridazine
tizanidine
venlafaxine
voriconazole
ziprasidone
zolmitriptan

Infusion rates

Nitroglycerin infusion rates

Determine the infusion rate in ml/hr using the ordered dose and the concentration of the drug solution.

Dose (mcg/min)	25 mg/250 ml (100 mcg/ml)	50 mg/250 ml (200 mcg/ml)	100 mg/250 ml (400 mcg/ml)
5	3	2	1
10	6	3	2
20	12	6	3
30	18	9	5
40	24	12	6
50	30	15	8
60	36	18	9
70	42	21	10
80	48	24	12
90	54	27	14
100	60	30	15
150	90	45	23
200	120	60	30

Dobutamine infusion rates

Mix 250 mg in 250 ml of D$_5$W (1,000 mcg/ml). Determine the infusion rate in ml/hr using the ordered dose and the patient's weight in pounds or kilograms.

Dose (mcg/kg/min)	lb 88 / kg 40	99 / 45	110 / 50	121 / 55	132 / 60	143 / 65	154 / 70	165 / 75	176 / 80	187 / 85	198 / 90	209 / 95	220 / 100	231 / 105	242 / 110
2.5	6	7	8	8	9	10	11	11	12	13	14	14	15	16	17
5	12	14	15	17	18	20	21	23	24	26	27	29	30	32	33
7.5	18	20	23	25	27	29	32	34	36	38	41	43	45	47	50
10	24	27	30	33	36	39	42	45	48	51	54	57	60	63	66
12.5	30	34	38	41	45	49	53	56	60	64	68	71	75	79	83
15	36	41	45	50	54	59	63	68	72	77	81	86	90	95	99
20	48	54	60	66	72	78	84	90	96	102	108	114	120	126	132
25	60	68	75	83	90	98	105	113	120	128	135	143	150	158	165
30	72	81	90	99	108	117	126	135	144	153	162	171	180	189	198
35	84	95	105	116	126	137	147	158	168	179	189	200	210	221	231
40	96	108	120	132	144	156	168	180	192	204	216	228	240	252	264

(continued)

Dopamine infusion rates

Mix 400 mg in 250 ml of D$_5$W (1,600 mcg/ml). Determine the infusion rate in ml/hr using the ordered dose and the patient's weight in pounds or kilograms.

Dose (mcg/kg/min)	lb 88	99	110	121	132	143	154	165	176	187	198	209	220	231
	kg 40	45	50	55	60	65	70	75	80	85	90	95	100	105
2.5	4	4	5	5	6	6	7	7	8	8	8	9	9	10
5	8	8	9	10	11	12	13	14	15	16	17	18	19	20
7.5	11	13	14	15	17	18	20	21	23	24	25	27	28	30
10	15	17	19	21	23	24	26	28	30	32	34	36	38	39
12.5	19	21	23	26	28	30	33	35	38	40	42	45	47	49
15	23	25	28	31	34	37	39	42	45	48	51	53	56	59
20	30	34	38	41	45	49	53	56	60	64	68	71	75	79
25	38	42	47	52	56	61	66	70	75	80	84	89	94	98
30	45	51	56	62	67	73	79	84	90	96	101	107	113	118
35	53	59	66	72	79	85	92	98	105	112	118	125	131	138
40	60	68	75	83	90	98	105	113	120	128	135	143	150	158
45	68	76	84	93	101	110	118	127	135	143	152	160	169	177
50	75	84	94	103	113	122	131	141	150	159	169	178	188	197

Nitroprusside infusion rates

Mix 50 mg in 250 ml of D$_5$W (200 mcg/ml). Determine the infusion rate in ml/hr using the ordered dose and the patient's weight in pounds or kilograms.

Dose (mcg/ kg/ min)	lb 88	99	110	121	132	143	154	165	176	187	198	209	220	231	242
	kg 40	45	50	55	60	65	70	75	80	85	90	95	100	105	110
0.3	4	4	5	5	5	6	6	7	7	8	8	9	9	9	10
0.5	6	7	8	8	9	10	11	11	12	13	14	14	15	16	17
1	12	14	15	17	18	20	21	23	24	26	27	29	30	32	33
1.5	18	20	23	25	27	29	32	34	36	38	41	43	45	47	50
2	24	27	30	33	36	39	42	45	48	51	54	57	60	63	66
3	36	41	45	50	54	59	63	68	72	77	81	86	90	95	99
4	48	54	60	66	72	78	84	90	96	102	108	114	120	126	132
5	60	68	75	83	90	98	105	113	120	128	135	143	150	158	165
6	72	81	90	99	108	117	126	135	144	153	162	171	180	189	198
7	84	95	105	116	126	137	147	158	168	179	189	200	210	221	231
8	96	108	120	132	144	156	168	180	192	204	216	228	240	252	264
9	108	122	135	149	162	176	189	203	216	230	243	257	270	284	297
10	120	135	150	165	180	195	210	225	240	255	270	285	300	315	330

Dangerous laboratory test values

The abnormal laboratory test values listed below require immediate intervention.

Test	Low value	Possible causes	High value	Possible causes
Ammonia	< 15 mcg/dl	Renal failure	> 50 mcg/dl	Severe hepatic disease
Calcium, serum	< 7 mg/dl	Vitamin D or parathyroid hormone deficiency	> 12 mg/dl	Hyperparathyroidism
Carbon dioxide and bicarbonate, blood	< 10 mEq/L	Complex pattern of metabolic and respiratory factors	> 40 mEq/L	Complex pattern of metabolic and respiratory factors
Creatinine, serum	Not applicable	Not applicable	> 4 mg/dl	Renal failure
Creatine kinase (CK-MB)	Not applicable	Not applicable	> 5%	Acute MI
D-dimer, serum or CSF	Not applicable	Not applicable	> 250 mcg/ml	Disseminated intravascular coagulation (DIC), PE, thrombosis, subarachnoid hemorrhage (CSF only), secondary fibrinolysis
Glucose, blood	< 40 mg/dl	Excess insulin	> 300 mg/dl	Diabetes
Hemoglobin	< 8 g/dl	Hemorrhage, vitamin B_{12} or iron deficiency	>18 g/dl	COPD
INR	Not applicable	Not applicable	> 3	DIC, anticoagulation

Test	Low value	Possible causes	High value	Possible causes
Paco$_2$	< 20 mm Hg	Complex pattern of metabolic and respiratory factors	> 70 mm Hg	Complex pattern of metabolic and respiratory factors
Pao$_2$	< 50 mm Hg	Complex pattern of metabolic and respiratory factors		Complex pattern of metabolic and respiratory factors
pH, blood	< 7.2	Complex pattern of metabolic and respiratory factors	> 7.6	Complex pattern of metabolic and respiratory factors
Platelet count	< 50,000/mm^3	Bone marrow suppression	> 50,000/mm^3	Leukemia, reaction to acute bleeding
Potassium, serum	< 3 mEq/L	Vomiting and diarrhea, diuretic therapy	> 6 mEq/L	Renal impairment
PT	Not applicable	Not applicable	> 14 sec (> 20 sec for patient taking warfarin)	Anticoagulant therapy, anticoagulation factor deficiency
PTT	Not applicable	Not applicable	> 40 sec (> 70 sec for patient taking heparin)	Anticoagulation factor deficiency
Sodium, serum	< 120 mEq/L	Diuretic therapy	> 160 mEq/L	Dehydration
WBC count	< 2,000/mm^3	Bone marrow suppression	> 20,000/mm^3	Leukemia
WBC count, CSF	Not applicable	Not applicable	> 10/mm^3	Meningitis, encephalitis

Index

A

Abbreviations, v-vii
Abdominal distention, neostigmine for, 110
Abdominal infection, internal. *See* Intra-abdominal infection.
Abdominal surgery
    dalteparin for, 40
    enoxaparin for, 53
Abelcet, 10
Ability, 13
Abortion
    ertapenem for, 56
    mifepristone for, 103-104
    oxytocin for, 118
Abreva, 47
Accolate, 158-159
AccuNeb, 3-4
Accupril, 132-133
Acephen, 1-2
Aceta, 1-2
Acetadote, 2
Acetaminophen toxicity, acetylcysteine for, 2
acetylsalicylic acid, 13
Achromycin, 147-148
Acid indigestion. *See also* Gastroesophageal reflux disease.
    calcium carbonate for, 23
    magnesium salts for, 95
    sodium bicarbonate for, 142

Aciduria, methylmalonic, cyanocobalamin for, 39
Aciphex, 133-134
Acne, tretinoin for, 153
Acquired immunodeficiency syndrome. *See* Human immunodeficiency virus infection.
Acromegaly, bromocriptine for, 20
Acticort, 78
Actidose, 2
Actidose-Aqua, 2
Actinic keratosis
    diclofenac for, 43
    fluorouracil for, 65
Actiq, 62
Activase, 6
Actonel, 136
Actos, 125
Acute coronary syndrome, clopidogrel for, 36
Acute lymphocytic leukemia
    methotrexate for, 99
    vincristine for, 158
Adalat, 111
Adalat CC, 111
Adapin, 49
Adenocard, 3
Adoxa, 49-50
Adrenalin, 54
Adrenalin Chloride, 54
adrenaline, 54

Adrenal insufficiency
    fludrocortisone for, 64
    hydrocortisone for, 78
Adrenogenital syndrome, fludrocortisone for, 64
Adrucil, 65
Adsorbocarpine, 124-125
Advil, 79
Aerolate, 148
Agenerase, 12
Agitation
    lorazepam for, 93
    ziprasidone for, 160
A-hydroCort, 77-78
AIDS. *See* Human immunodeficiency virus infection.
AK-Dex, 42
AKTob, 151
Alavert, 93
Alcohol dependence, naltrexone for, 108
Alcohol withdrawal
    chlordiazepoxide for, 31
    clorazepate for, 37
    oxazepam for, 116
Aldactone, 142
Aldomet, 99
Aleve, 108-109
Alinia, 111
Alka-Mints, 22-23
Allegra, 63
Allerdryl, 45-46
Allergic conjunctivitis
    dexamethasone for, 42
    epinastine for, 53